AF389175

3D Printed Materials Dentistry

3D Printed Materials Dentistry

Editor

Kathrin Becker

MDPI • Basel • Beijing • Wuhan • Barcelona • Belgrade • Manchester • Tokyo • Cluj • Tianjin

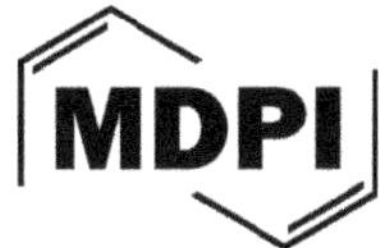

Editor
Kathrin Becker
University Hospital Dusseldorf
Germany

Editorial Office
MDPI
St. Alban-Anlage 66
4052 Basel, Switzerland

This is a reprint of articles from the Special Issue published online in the open access journal *Applied Sciences* (ISSN 2076-3417) (available at: https://www.mdpi.com/journal/applsci/special_issues/3D_Printed_Materials_Dentistry).

For citation purposes, cite each article independently as indicated on the article page online and as indicated below:

LastName, A.A.; LastName, B.B.; LastName, C.C. Article Title. *Journal Name* **Year**, *Volume Number*, Page Range.

ISBN 978-3-0365-6888-1 (Hbk)
ISBN 978-3-0365-6889-8 (PDF)

Contents

About the Editor

Kathrin Becker

Kathrin Becker studied Dentistry at the University of Greifswald and Gottingen (Germany), as well as Applied Computer Science (Bachelor and Master of Science) at the University of Gottingen. Her master's degree was awarded with distinction, and she was awarded with a short-term research scholarship at the University of Pittsburgh (USA). She received her Doctorate (magna cum laude) from the University of Dusseldorf (2014). She performed her specialty training in orthodontics from 2014–2018 at the same university under the leadership of Prof. Dr. D. Drescher. She completed a Habilitation in Dentistry and Maxillofacial Medicine in 2019. Since 2021, she has been the Assistant Medical Director at the Department for Orthodontics (University Hospital Dusseldorf). Currently, she is member in various committees from international societies (Osteology expert council, EAO congress committee, EAO junior committee, and Osteology Scientific Review Board), Editorial Board member (*Journal of Clinical Periodontology*, *Clinical Oral Implants Research*, and *Clinical Oral Investigations*), and Editor-in-Chief of the Wiley and Sons Ltd. *Journal Clinical and Experimental Dental Research*. She has published 90 peer reviewed articles and has been awarded with research prizes: Osteology (2019), Young Scientists Award (2014), and Publons Reviewer Award (1× 2019, 2× 2020), and she has been selected by the University of Dusseldorf for the Selma Meyer Mentoring Programme and the Academic Career Development Programme. Her research interests comprise but are not limited to skeletal anchorage, application of 3D-imging in dentistry, e-learning in dentistry, and micro-computed tomography.

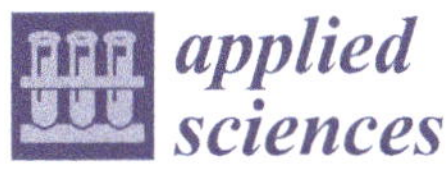

Editorial

3D-Printed Materials Dentistry

Kathrin Becker

Department of Orthodontics, University Hospital Dusseldorf, 40225 Dusseldorf, Germany; kathrin.becker@med.uni-duesseldorf.de; Tel.: +49-211-8118160

Citation: Becker, K. 3D-Printed Materials Dentistry. *Appl. Sci.* **2023**, *13*, 457. https://doi.org/10.3390/app13010457

Received: 23 December 2022
Accepted: 27 December 2022
Published: 29 December 2022

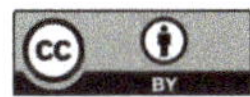

This editorial focuses on the Special Issue on 3D-printed materials in dentistry. The articles of this Special Issue cover a wide range of applications in the dental field. They range from applications in the clinical workplace to in vitro investigations on the impact of postcuring and storage time on accuracy and precision measurements to the indirect transfer of orthodontic brackets, as well as the application of 3D printing in dental education. Five out of eleven research papers deal with applications of 3D printing in orthodontics, one study presents a 3D-printed fitting system for FFP2 masks which were applied during the COVID-19 pandemic, while the remaining one addresses applications in prosthodontics and restorative dentistry.

In orthodontics, 3D printing is becoming increasingly popular. It allows to create individualized appliances, to perform different treatment tasks at the same time, and much more [1].

The article by Küffer et al. [2] demonstrates a digital workflow for producing highly individualized, skeletally borne 3D-designed appliances for the upper and the lower jaw. As orthodontic mini-implants providing skeletal anchorage are often inserted using templates, the article also presents typical designs for insertion guides. Additionally, it highlights potential sources of errors within the digital workflow that are especially relevant to clinicians in their daily practice.

The article by Kirschner et al. [3] addresses the question of whether steam autoclaving impacts on the biomechanical properties of 3D-printed insertion guides. Autoclaving is necessary as the guides may be in contact with blood during orthodontic implant placements. The study compared two autoclaving cycles and different resin/printer combinations. For the protocol using a lower temperature and a longer autoclaving time, no biomechanical alterations could be observed, whereas in some groups, significant difference were noted for the faster autoclaving protocol at an increased temperature.

The article by Ihssen et al. [4] investigated whether the socket height of 3D-printed casts used to thermoform aligners has an impact on the aligner thickness and homogeneity. Thicker aligners would apply higher forces to the teeth, and varying thickness values might lead to inhomogeneous force applications across the aligners. Indeed, the study demonstrated that increased socket height was associated with thinner and more homogeneous aligners. Additionally, in all groups, the thickness values were highest at the incisal surfaces, and they were the lowest at the facial aspects, especially at the cervical margins. Future clinical studies are needed to assess the impact of local variation in the aligner thickness on the local force application and thus on treatment's success.

The article by Jungbauer et al. [5] compared two 3D-printed bracket transfer trays with different shore hardnesses and assessed whether the crowding of the incisors impacts on the accuracy of indirect bracket transfer. Additionally, the workflow was tested using two different methods, i.e., intraoral scanning and Micro-CT, whereby intraoral scanning was inferior as the shape of the brackets was very different from that of the reference. The study found minor linear deviations for the indirect bracket transfer, whereas angular deviations and deviations in the torque reached values that were above the limits specified by the American Board of Orthodontists. Finally, the deviations were more pronounced for crowded teeth.

Mieszala et al. [6] proposed the fabrication of Polymer Polyether Ether Ketone (PEEK) transpalatal arches designed in a CAD process. The forces and moments of two transpalatal arch designs were within a range that appears to be clinically useful for expansion or for anchorage purposes. However, their clinical applicability is still limited as the PEEK arches cannot be activated intraorally. Furthermore, there is also a lack of clinical studies proving their applicability in clinical settings.

Vichi et al. [7] focused on infection control during COVID-19 pandemic. They designed a mask fitter to ensure proper fit of FFP2 masks. While no data are available on the efficacy of this device, they reported a high satisfaction of staff members with the novel mask fitting system.

The article focusing on dental education by Lugassy et al. [8] described the fabrication of multi-colored teeth to train students in Class I preparations of molars. The study demonstrated low reliability in evaluations of undergraduate students given by staff for conventional plastic molars, whereas moderate to good reliability was found for the multicolored 3D-printed teeth. Thus, it was concluded that the multicolored teeth can provide a more objective evaluation of the students' performance in cavity preparation.

The article by Lin et al. [9] focused on the dimensional stability of 3D-printed casts obtained using digital light processing (DLP) or stereolithography (SLA). While no shrinkage was noted in the first two weeks for DLP and SLA groups, a significant contraction was noted from two to six weeks.

The article of Doh et al. [10] focused on the dimensional changes during the postcuring of 3D-printed denture bases. They found that the dimensional changes increased with postcuring times of 15–60 min, and that accuracy was higher when no prior removal of support structures had been performed.

The article by Lüchtenborg et al. [11] outlined the potential applications of fused filament fabrication (FFF) printing in dentistry. Despite FFF was reported to exhibit a reduced accuracy compared to that of other 3D printing technologies, this technology was reported to be a promising and cost-efficient alternative for the in-house production of digitally designed models, trays, or prototypes for denture try-ins.

The article by Çakmak et al. [12] investigated the impact of the 3D printing layer thickness on the trueness and margin quality of interim dental crowns in comparison to that of milled PMMA crowns. They demonstrated that milled PMMA crowns had the highest margin quality, while printed crowns with a layer thickness of 20μm and 100μm had the lowest. They also found that the trueness and marginal quality of the 3D-printed interim crowns were influenced by the printing layer thickness. Trueness of milled crowns was reported to be superior compared to 100 μm printed crowns, and margin quality was also highest for milled crowns.

In summary, the publications of this Special Issue reflect the multitude of areas in which 3D printing technologies can be applied to dentistry at present, and they also outline future avenues for novel research projects. As the majority of studies were performed in vitro, this Special Issue might also stimulate future clinical studies and systematic reviews of the existing literature.

Acknowledgments: The editor would like to acknowledge the authors for their valuable contributions and the referees for their fruitful and critical suggestions which led to the high quality of the manuscripts and the entire Special Issue.

Conflicts of Interest: The author declares no conflict of interest.

References

1. Tarraf, N.E.; Ali, D.M. Present and the future of digital orthodontics. *Semin. Orthod.* **2018**, *24*, 376–385. [CrossRef]
2. Küffer, M.; Drescher, D.; Becker, K. Application of the Digital Workflow in Orofacial Orthopedics and Orthodontics: Printed Appliances with Skeletal Anchorage. *Appl. Sci.* **2022**, *12*, 3820. [CrossRef]
3. Kirschner, A.; David, S.; Brunello, G.; Keilig, L.; Drescher, D.; Bourauel, C.; Becker, K. Impact of Steam Autoclaving on the Mechanical Properties of 3D-Printed Resins Used for Insertion Guides in Orthodontics and Implant Dentistry. *Appl. Sci.* **2022**, *12*, 6195. [CrossRef]

4. Ihssen, B.; Kerberger, R.; Rauch, N.; Drescher, D.; Becker, K. Impact of Dental Model Height on Thermoformed PET-G Aligner Thickness—An In Vitro Micro-CT Study. *Appl. Sci.* **2021**, *11*, 6674. [CrossRef]
5. Jungbauer, R.; Breunig, J.; Schmid, A.; Hüfner, M.; Kerberger, R.; Rauch, N.; Becker, K. Transfer Accuracy of Two 3D Printed Trays for Indirect Bracket Bonding—An In Vitro Pilot Study. *Appl. Sci.* **2021**, *11*, 6013. [CrossRef]
6. Mieszala, C.; Schmidt, J.G.; Becker, K.; Willmann, J.H.; Drescher, D. Digital Design of Different Transpalatal Arches Made of Polyether Ether Ketone (PEEK) and Determination of the Force Systems. *Appl. Sci.* **2022**, *12*, 1590. [CrossRef]
7. Vichi, A.; Balestra, D.; Goracci, C.; Radford, D.R.; Louca, C. The Mask Fitter, a Simple Method to Improve Medical Face Mask Adaptation Using a Customized 3D-Printed Frame during COVID-19: A Survey on Users' Acceptability in Clinical Dentistry. *Appl. Sci.* **2022**, *12*, 8921. [CrossRef]
8. Lugassy, D.; Awad, M.; Shely, A.; Davidovitch, M.; Pilo, R.; Brosh, T. 3D-Printed Teeth with Multicolored Layers as a Tool for Evaluating Cavity Preparation by Dental Students. *Appl. Sci.* **2021**, *11*, 6406. [CrossRef]
9. Lin, L.; Granatelli, J.; Alifui-Segbaya, F.; Drake, L.; Smith, D.; Ahmed, K. A Proposed In Vitro Methodology for Assessing the Accuracy of Three-Dimensionally Printed Dental Models and the Impact of Storage on Dimensional Stability. *Appl. Sci.* **2021**, *11*, 5994. [CrossRef]
10. Doh, R.-M.; Kim, J.-E.; Nam, N.-E.; Shin, S.-H.; Lim, J.-H.; Shim, J.-S. Evaluation of Dimensional Changes during Postcuring of a Three-Dimensionally Printed Denture Base According to the Curing Time and the Time of Removal of the Support Structure: An In Vitro Study. *Appl. Sci.* **2021**, *11*, 10000. [CrossRef]
11. Lüchtenborg, J.; Burkhardt, F.; Nold, J.; Rothlauf, S.; Wesemann, C.; Pieralli, S.; Wemken, G.; Witkowski, S.; Spies, B. Implementation of Fused Filament Fabrication in Dentistry. *Appl. Sci.* **2021**, *11*, 6444. [CrossRef]
12. Çakmak, G.; Cuellar, A.R.; Donmez, M.B.; Schimmel, M.; Abou-Ayash, S.; Lu, W.E.; Yilmaz, B. Effect of Printing Layer Thickness on the Trueness and Margin Quality of 3D-Printed Interim Dental Crowns. *Appl. Sci.* **2021**, *11*, 9246. [CrossRef]

applied
sciences

Communication

Application of the Digital Workflow in Orofacial Orthopedics and Orthodontics: Printed Appliances with Skeletal Anchorage

Maximilian Küffer *, Dieter Drescher and Kathrin Becker

Department of Orthodontics, University Clinic Düsseldorf, Moorenstrasse 5, 40225 Düsseldorf, Germany; drescher@med.uni-duesseldorf.de (D.D.); kathrin.becker@med.uni-duesseldorf.de (K.B.)
* Correspondence: kueffer@med.uni-duesseldorf.de

Abstract: As digital workflows are gaining popularity, novel treatment options have also arisen in orthodontics. By using selective laser melting (SLM), highly customized 3D-printed appliances can be manufactured and combined with preformed components. When combined with temporary anchorage devices (TADs), the advantages of the two approaches can be merged, which might improve treatment efficacy, versatility, and patient comfort. This article summarizes state-of-the-art technologies and digital workflows to design and install 3D-printed skeletally anchored orthodontic appliances. The advantages and disadvantages of digital workflows are critically discussed, and examples for the clinical application of mini-implant and mini-plate borne appliances are demonstrated.

Keywords: digital workflow; orthodontic; skeletal anchorage; temporary anchorage device; 3D printing; printed appliance; metal printing

Citation: Küffer, M.; Drescher, D.; Becker, K. Application of the Digital Workflow in Orofacial Orthopedics and Orthodontics: Printed Appliances with Skeletal Anchorage. *Appl. Sci.* **2022**, *12*, 3820. https://doi.org/10.3390/app12083820

Academic Editor: Andrea Scribante

Received: 28 February 2022
Accepted: 6 April 2022
Published: 10 April 2022

Publisher's Note: MDPI stays neutral with regard to jurisdictional claims in published maps and institutional affiliations.

1. Introduction

Digital technologies, such as 3D scanning and printing, have expanded the range of treatment options in various medical disciplines in recent years [1–5]. In dentistry, a wide range of possible implementations have been reported across specialties, including the fields of orofacial orthopedics and orthodontics [6]. In contemporary orthodontics, scanning dental arches for metric analyses or the creation of digital set-ups are routinely performed. A relatively new application is the design and clinical application of individual metal-printed orthodontic appliances [7]. Especially in complex cases, where conventional techniques and preformed devices do not fulfill all requirements, individualized 3D-designed and printed appliances may be advantageous [7,8]. In addition, appliances created using a digital workflow are reported to offer many advantages in terms of patient comfort, treatment efficacy, and predictability [7,8].

As every orthodontic (and orthopedic) force is associated with a reactive force of equal magnitude, orthodontic treatment success necessitates sufficient anchorage to avoid side effects, including undesired tooth movement of dental anchorage units [9,10]. Therefore, orthodontic anchorage is a term for all measures preventing those reactive forces and moments [11]. Typically, either teeth (dental units) or extraoral attachments are used. Extra-anchorage can be achieved by integrating the bone into the resistance unit by means of so-called temporary anchorage devices (TADs). This concept is called skeletal anchorage, and it gained popularity in recent years owing to a reduction in side effects and increased treatment efficacy [8–10,12–17]. Among the TADs, orthodontic mini-implants are frequently employed due to their ease of application and the favorable cost–benefit ratio [18,19].

In the upper jaw, the anterior palate proved to be the most favorable insertion site with the highest survival rates [15,20,21]. In the mandible, however, mini-implants usually have to be inserted into the alveolar ridge [22–24], where failure rates range from 14% to 16% [25–27]. The lower success rates were mainly attributed to the reduced bone quality and the proximity to the dental roots. In addition, a risk of root contact or even penetration exists [25,26]. Since mini-implants are inserted between the roots, the extent of possible orthodontic tooth movement is implicitly limited. Mini-implants inserted into the mandibular buccal shelf did not gain much acceptance in most of the countries because of their very low survival rates [27], despite their advantage not to limit tooth movements. Alternatively, the chin below the dental roots was identified as a possible insertion site due to its high bone quantity and quality. Nonetheless, mini-implants are not well-suited for the area, and thus special mini-plates, such as the Mentoplate, were developed [28,29]. These plates can be fixed to the bone using regular osteosynthesis screws, but require a slightly more invasive surgical procedure for insertion and removal, when compared with mini-implants.

TAD-borne appliances are regarded as "non-compliance" devices as patients only need to keep them clean, but are not requested to wear them for a certain amount of hours (they have to wear them 24 h/day) [30]. These appliances also permit longer time intervals between appointments and hence a reduction of the overall chair-time [10,12,31].

The application of digital workflows to design and manufacture TAD-borne appliances appears to be particularly promising. The placement of the mini-implants can be planned, which allows the identification of the optimal insertion position based on digital models and, optionally, using radiographs. Utilizing printed insertion guides [32] or the appliance itself [33] allows for implant insertion and appliance installation in one appointment. Owing to the precise fitting, the risk of screw overloading, and therefore the risk of implant failure, can be reduced [34,35]. However, digital workflows rely on the skills and experience of the operator, and pitfalls exist that can limit the advantages of the digital workflow.

The present article describes a fully digital workflow for the creation of TAD-borne metal printed appliances in orthodontics and orofacial orthopedics. Accordingly, some of the most common printing techniques and materials, possible advantages and disadvantages, and potential sources of error are critically discussed.

2. Digital Workflow: From Intraoral Scan to the Printable Data

2.1. Data Acquisition

A fundamental basis for the digital design of orthodontic appliances is gathering information regarding the intraoral situation including teeth, alveolar ridge, and soft tissues. This can be achieved using intraoral scanning or by employing digitized conventional plaster casts. Some studies found the intraoral scan to be more time-consuming than conventional methods [36,37], whereas others did not observe any significant difference [38]. This might indicate that the practitioners' level of experience could have a major impact on time efficacy. In addition, several studies underlined a sufficient accuracy and precision of intraoral scans for orthodontic purposes [36–39]. Further advantages of digital impressions compared to conventional ones include gains in comfort for the patient and a reduced amount of laboratory waste [7,8,37,39].

Data can be stored in various formats. Nonetheless, the Standard Tessellation Language (STL) format was shown to be the smallest common denominator for 3D data exchange between devices and software programs [8,36].

2.2. Digital Appliance Design

In order to design and manufacture an appliance, the intraoral scan generally requires further processing, including mesh repair, hole filling, and removal of invalid data. Usually, a base is added to the dental arch to form a model (Figure 1).

Software tools that enable digital planning range from open-source over freeware to proprietary solutions. Currently, there is great variability in software complexity, sometimes necessitating a steep learning curve.

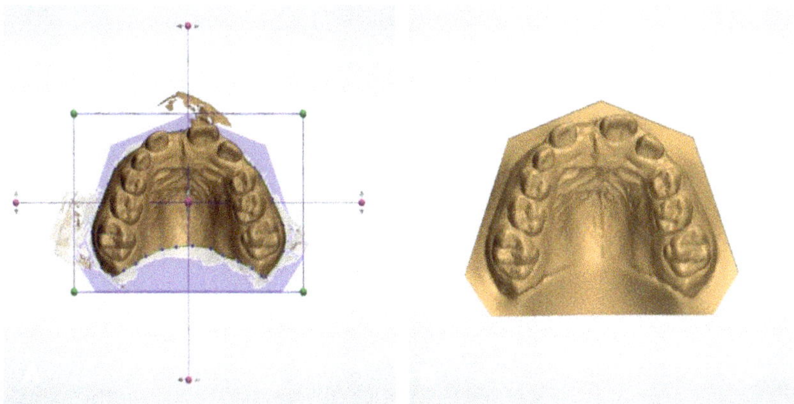

Figure 1. Processing of an intraoral scan to a digital model: (**A**) Removal of noise at the edges, and virtual placement within a digital socket. (**B**) Completed digital model (software: Appliance Designer, 3Shape).

The computer-aided design of the orthodontic appliances enables the planning of all steps, including the positioning of orthodontic mini-implants (Figure 2) or osteosynthesis screws and the position of shells or attachments. Moreover, functional elements can be adapted, for example, by modifying their shape, adjusting the inclination and tilt of gliding mechanisms, or manipulating the expansion of orthodontic screws. Simulation of planned tooth movements is also possible, enabling clinicians to oversee and predict treatment outcomes. Additionally, communication with technicians is simplified. Groups of teeth required to move in a specific direction can be connected to active elements of the appliance, and comparison of actual with predicted tooth movements enables validation (Figure 3).

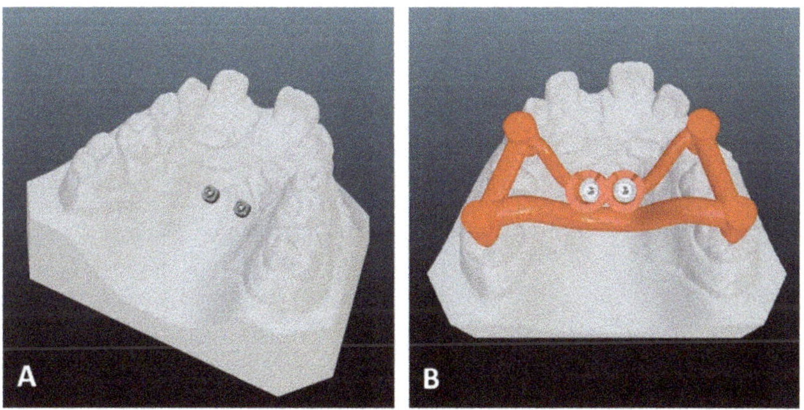

Figure 2. (**A**) Virtual implant planning on a digital model. (**B**) Virtual design of an insertion guide, that can be 3D-printed (software: Blender, Blender Foundation).

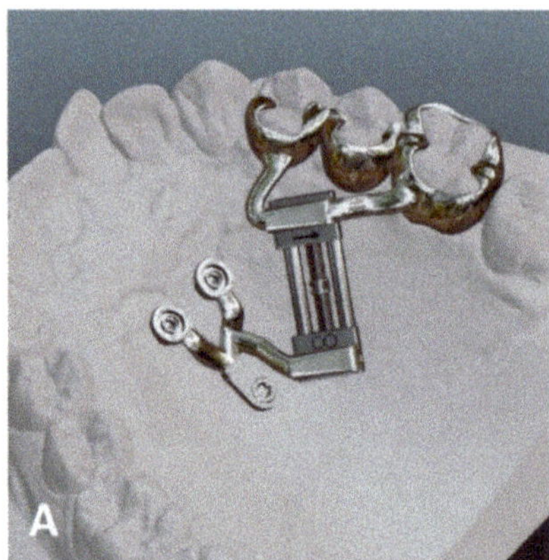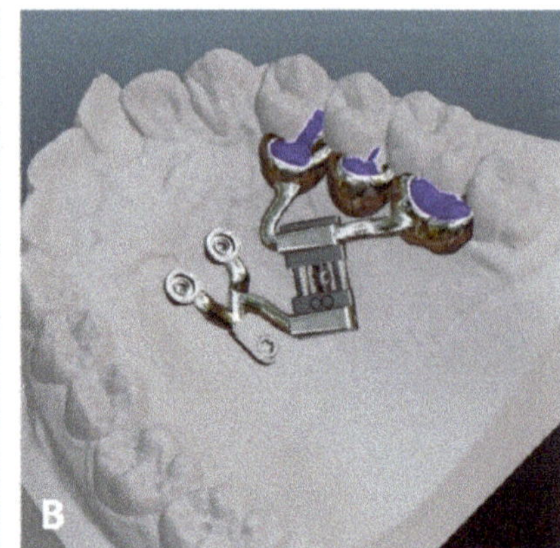

Figure 3. (**A**) Customized active element connected to implants and teeth. (**B**) Simulated activation with estimated movement of teeth (blue) (software: Blender, Blender Foundation).

When skeletal anchorage is employed, an accurate fit of the digitally planned appliance is fundamental to avoid overloading of the orthodontic implants. One option is to perform data acquisition after implant insertion. Sometimes, scanners show problems recognizing the metallic implants, which can be improved using scanning spray or scan bodies [40]. The other option is to insert the mini-implants upon digital planning through guides and utilize the planned position for the appliance design. Digitally planned insertion guides allow implant and appliance insertion within the same visit [40–43] (Figure 2). This can also be achieved by using so-called *Direct Screws*, which are inserted after the adhesive bond of the appliance onto the teeth [33]. As the appliances themselves serve as an insertion aid, no additional guide is needed. When installing a printed *Mentoplate* with supra-constructions for orthodontic tooth movement, a guided insertion is mandatory to precisely achieve the planned position and ensure the fit of supra-construction and teeth.

Digital positioning of (mini-)implants is an already established process in prosthodontic and orthodontic treatments. For insertion of orthodontic screws in the anterior palate, 3D radiographic images are oftentimes not needed. Nonetheless, radiographs can help to estimate the available bone supply [40,44], and they are indicated in case of palatially displaced teeth, limited bone supply, or pathologies, including clefts (Figure 4). Lateral cephalograms provided a sufficient approximation when compared to cone-beam computed tomography (CBCT) for most of the patients [41,45,46]. In case of displaced teeth, patients with craniofacial anomalies, or in case of insufficient bone height visible on a cephalogram, optimal insertion sites and angles can be identified with the help of 3D radiographs [46]. In case of impacted teeth, the optimal vector for force application may also be incorporated in the digital design based on the information from CBCT [12] (Figure 4B).

The digital design of mini-plates for the chin bone requires a CBCT to enable an accurate fit. The segmented chin may be matched with an intraoral scan to create an appliance with transmucosal extensions. As root localization is clearly visible in the CBCT, damage of (unerupted) teeth or roots during screw insertion can be avoided. It is also possible to shape the surface of the bottom of the device in perfect match with the superficial structure of the bone, ensuring wide and evenly flat contact that might prevent side effects.

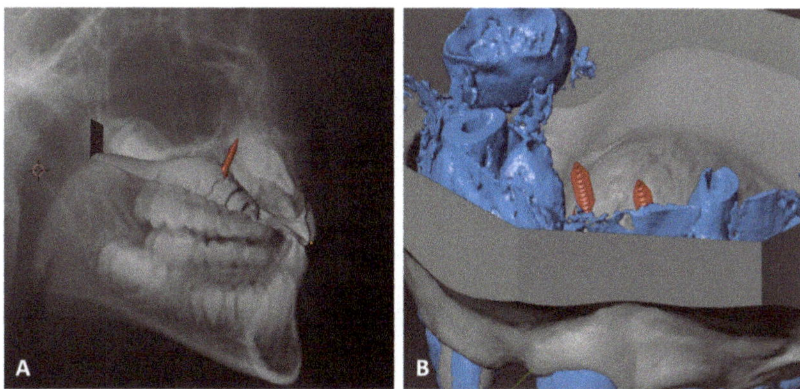

Figure 4. (**A**) Superimposed lateral ceph radiograph for the planning of implant placement. (**B**) CBCT can aid implant placement planning in more complex cases (software: Blender, Blender Foundation).

If clinicians do not design the appliance themselves, the manufacturing laboratory can send the digital draft of the designed appliance back to the clinician, enabling an easy and fast way to revise it, approve it, and communicate desired changes [7,8,47]. Whereas conventionally manufactured appliances would have to be reproduced in case of breakage or improper fit, digital appliances can be reprinted based on the stored data [7], unless they have already been activated in a non-reproducible way.

2.3. Data Preparation for 3D Printing

Since the printing of three-dimensional structures is achieved by adding and joining two-dimensional layers, it is possible to construct very complex and individual structures [48,49]. Printing potential has very few limitations, making preformed pieces just under certain indications necessary. Small parts with internal hollow spaces and pieces with very high requirements regarding the accuracy of fit, such as tubes, elements with internal mechanics, or orthodontic screws, cannot be printed, but can be added by welding them to the printed framework of the appliance. The possibility to create an appliance adapted to the specific intraoral conditions of a patient, almost independent from standardized preformed parts, also allows manufacturing of customized devices for complex and challenging treatment needs [7,47].

The materials used to print the insertion guides for orthodontic implants have to be biocompatible and sterilizable [40]. A precise fit of the insertion tool within the guide's sleeves is needed to achieve an accurate insertion of the implants. Only minor discrepancies, especially in the vertical direction, are tolerable [41]. Vertical control can be improved by using insertion instruments facilitating vertical control [40].

3. 3D Printing Technologies for Orthodontic Appliances

Orthodontic appliances with skeletal anchorage require a metal framework and are usually manufactured by selective laser melting and sintering (SLM/SLS). This additive manufacturing is a kind of solid freeform fabrication and belongs to the powder bed fusion techniques. Since the invention of selective laser sintering (SLS) in 1989 by Carl Deckard, there has been constant progress in the further development of this technique. Using different sources of energy and powdered materials, SLS and SLM can be applied to almost every material melted by laser radiation which solidifies while cooling down, thus making it one of the most versatile additive manufacturing techniques [48,50]. In this technique, a laser emitter moves over a bed of metal powder (e.g., CrCoW) which is heated minimally below its melting point. By tracing the modulated laser over the compacted powder, heat-fusible materials selectively melt in layers. Upon completion of a layer, the powder bed containing the structures being printed is lowered and new material is provided by rolling a thin coating of powder on top (Figure 5).

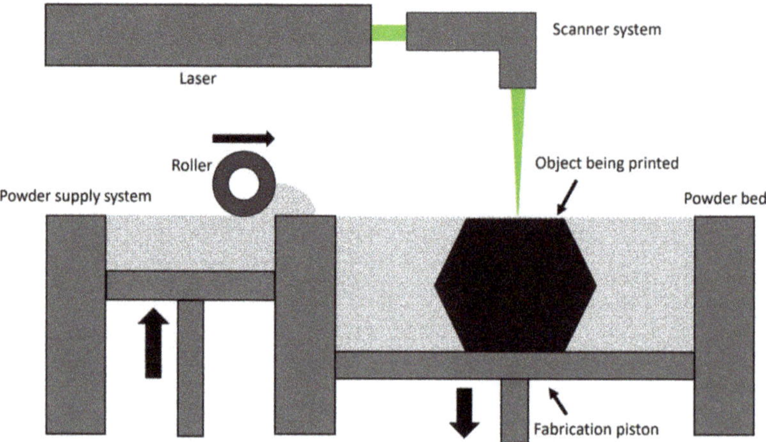

Figure 5. Scheme of SLM fabrication process.

Modern SLS can produce objects in layers with a thickness of 30–200 μm, depending on the particle size of the powder [49,50]. Once a structure is finished, the remaining powder must be brushed or blown off. Depending on the laser's power and the used material, the particles are sintered or fully melted together. In SLS, the emitted laser melts the grains' surface, while the core stays unaffected and solid. This partial melting allows for binding between the grains. Employing higher-powered lasers melts the grains fully to the core, resulting in homogenous structures, which solidify by cooling down [48]. Equipped with highly powered precision lasers, SLM improved many disadvantages of SLS, such as rough surfaces with high porosities and large shrink rates of the produced parts [48–50]. On the other hand, complete melting leads to higher surface tensions and therefore requires a smaller thickness of layers [48]. SLM-produced objects demonstrated high accuracy and precision in prosthodontic research, satisfying clinical requirements, sometimes surpassing other methods such as casting or milling [51–54].

Metal powders used for three-dimensional printing must fulfill all requirements regarding biocompatibility, thus allowing a safe mid- and long-term use in the oral environment. Therefore, alloys certified for oral application are commonly utilized for orthodontic purposes, among which, chromium-cobalt alloys [6,8,51,54,55] and titanium alloys for submucosal placements [48,50,55] are the most popular in orthodontics.

In the post-processing, the surface must be milled to remove all supporting structures as well as the rough outer oxide layer. Since SLS/SLM requires fewer supporting structures, post-processing is eased compared to other additive manufacturing procedures [49] (Figure 6A). If needed, preformed parts such as orthodontic screws, hooks for extraoral gears, or tubes can be added to the device by welding them to the framework (Figure 6B,C). Appliances designed with direct screws also require the matching thread to be welded onto the framework, because its co-axial construction is too complex to be printed.

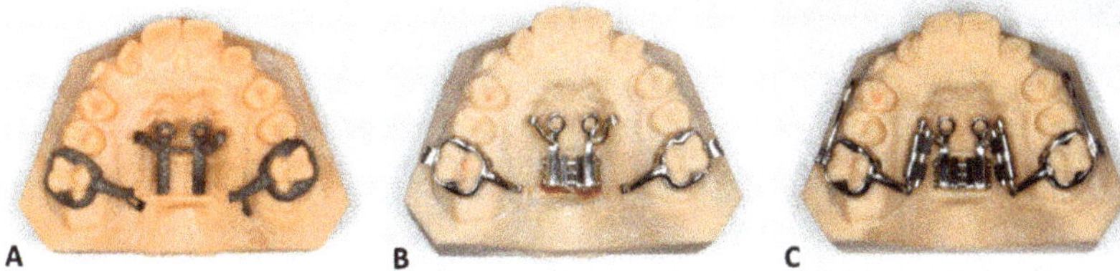

Figure 6. Post-processing of a 3D-printed appliance. (**A**) Unprocessed printed parts, (**B**) surface milled and polished, Jack screw and tubes welded to the appliance, (**C**) completed appliance for molar distalization and simultaneous face mask wear (hooks).

Auxiliary devices such as insertion guides or models are usually manufactured using printing resin materials. Depending on the purpose and the chosen resin, printing technologies can be divided into light curing and fused deposition modeling (FDM) [6,55]. Photosensitive resins can be printed using specific light-curing techniques called stereolithography (SLA), digital light processing (DLP), and photo jet (PJ). In SLA and DLP, objects are shaped by applying selective UV-light irradiation to a reservoir of liquid resin. The polymerized resin is attached to a platform that moves at defined distances away from the light source, resulting in an incremental shaping of objects similar to the SLM process. In contrast, in PJ technologies, photopolymers are sprayed onto a platform by a horizontally moving print head. The light curing occurs simultaneously through a UV-light-emitting lamp positioned at the print head. Posteriorly, the platform moves away on the Z-axis in the desired amount of layer thickness, shaping the object in incremental layers. In light-curing 3D printers, almost any kind of liquid photopolymers can be used. By applying PJ, printing composites of resins and ceramics is possible. In FDM, objects are shaped by heating thermoplastic materials up to their melting points and printing filaments in layers. Besides conventional thermoplastic materials, biological thermoplasts, such as polylactic acid, polycaprolactone, or acrylonitrile-butadiene-styrene, can be employed in FDM [6,55]. If the printed object will be employed in the oral cavity and may come in direct contact with blood, the material must be sterilized prior to usage and requires the respective certification. Commonly used materials for printed medical devices can be sterilized using ethylene oxide, e-beam, hydrogen peroxide, gamma radiation, or steam sterilization in an autoclave, depending on the chosen polymer [56–61] and the national legal requirements. Moreover, a high degree of biocompatibility must be ensured for materials used in the oral cavity, regarding a lack of cytotoxic, sensitizing, or irritational properties.

4. Sources of Error

Printed appliances show very high precision, good fit, and low error rates. Nonetheless, digital workflows and clinical implementation are complex and require specific operational knowledge and exact working methods.

Depending on the chosen workflow and appliance installation mode, there are possible sources of error to be considered. In case that all steps have been accurately performed, guided insertion enables accurate insertion and appliance fits. However, minor errors may accumulate, and in this case implants may show a certain degree of variance from their planned position, resulting in poor congruence and thus requiring an adjustment of the device's connectors before installation. Position variance may occur due to the plastic guide's flexibility, if too much pressure forces the drills into a false angulation, or if the time period between the intraoral scan and the appointment of appliance insertion has been too long. In the latter case, the insertion template and the appliance itself can show variation due to a patient's natural growth or a change in the stage of eruption and tooth position. If the inconsistency between the implants and the connector is too big, tension will be placed on the connection, resulting in patient discomfort, implant overload, and potential implant failure. Nonetheless, the connectors can be minimally widened by using a milling cutter. Additionally, the rigid printing alloys also allow a certain degree of bending, leading to the possibility of readjusting and correcting minor inaccuracies. According to clinical experience, implants inserted into the patient's palate before the scan without a stabilizing appliance may trigger the patients' tongues to press against the implants, resulting in manipulation and a possible loss of the implants.

Direct Screw-borne appliances that are fixed onto the teeth prior to the implant insertion usually do not bear the risk of screw overloading or improper fit, as minor angular deviations can be compensated by the appliance. Nonetheless, insertion of the screws through the incorporated guides can generate moments and forces on the whole appliance when locking the screws into the thread of the connector, especially in case of angular discrepancies. This could stress implants and adhesive connections. As a result, the implants may loosen, or the adhesive bonds may weaken. Therefore, maintaining a correct insertion angle is strongly recommended. Similar to conventional appliances, printed metal devices can be subject to fracture or loss of adhesive connections to the teeth. Whereas screw-retained devices can be removed temporarily for repair, fracture of the direct screw-borne appliances may necessitate exchange of the implants whenever no intraoral repair is possible.

5. Clinical Application

5.1. Temporary Anchorage Device-Borne Appliances

When skeletal anchorage is employed, the non-digital workflow consists of unguided implant insertion, followed by a conventional silicone molding with impression caps. Then, the appliance is manufactured based on a plastered model with laboratory analogs, mainly consisting of preformed components. Once finished, the appliance can be installed unless it does not fit properly.

In contrast, for skeletally anchored appliances manufactured using a digital workflow, the clinician can choose and alter the mode of installation. The appliance can be designed to be fastened onto formerly placed implants, or it can be installed simultaneously with the implants using an insertion guide for the implantation, or it can be attached to the teeth prior to the implantation (*Direct Screws*). In the latter case, the appliance itself serves as an insertion template [33].

Taking a closer look into the various options of implant installation helps with outlining the respective advantages and disadvantages.

A common way to place an implant-supported appliance into the oral cavity is to set the implants at their determined position using an insertion guide (Figure 7A,B). This ensures a perfect match with the printed appliance (Figure 7C). Fixing the appliance to its skeletal anchor requires a mechanism that locks the appliance on top of the implants and prevents rotations. If a fixation screw is used, adapting the appliance, or changing to a completely different device, is possible [33] (Figure 7D). The adhesive bond between the appliance and teeth occurs before the insertion of the fastening screws.

In case of *Direct Screws*, the appliance itself serves as the guide [33] (Figure 8). In this case, the practitioner adhesively attaches the appliance to the teeth and then uses the hole of the appliance's connectors as an insertion aid. This installation method can be advantageous because it eradicates a possible mismatch between implants and the appliance, and eliminates the need for an additional 3D-printed insertion guide.

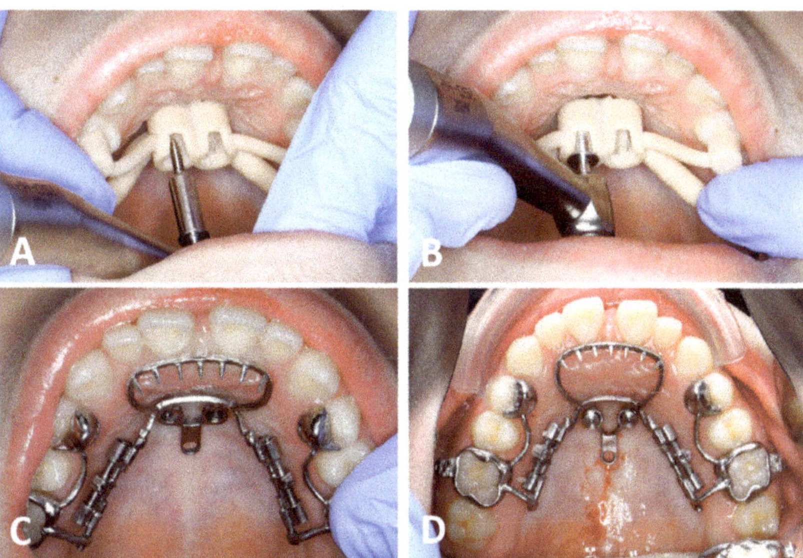

Figure 7. Appliance installation with guide: (**A**) Guided implantation. (**B**) Vertical control is achieved through a stop between the guide and the insertion tool. (**C**) Try-in on implants. (**D**) Appliance fastened on two implants by fixation screws.

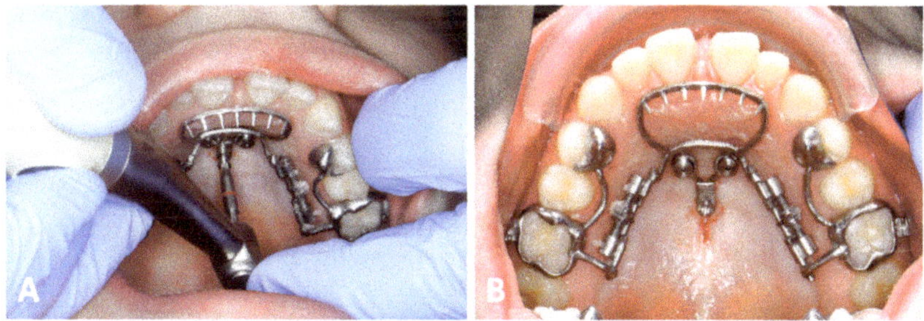

Figure 8. Direct screw insertion: (**A**) Implant placement with appliance itself serving as a guide. (**B**) Completed installation of the appliance from Figure 7 on two mini-implants (with fixation screws) and a posterior direct mini-implant inserted through the appliance itself.

When implant placement is performed prior to intraoral scanning, appliance installation is performed similar to conventional approaches. In case of immediate loading, one must consider that primary stability of the implants reduces within the first 4–6 weeks after insertion due to a loss of primary stability. Nonetheless, immediate loading of the implants has been reported to be not detrimental or even beneficial in terms of implant stability [62,63].

The molar coupling of digitally printed appliances can be achieved by means of printed shells or palatally attached tubes. These couplings do not penetrate the attached soft tissue and usually remain coronally to the interproximal contacts [64]. It may be speculated that this can lead to higher failure rates, which, however, can be reduced by etching the surface of the teeth and using an adhesive system instead of temporary cement. Additionally, no rubber-based separation of teeth is required prior to appliance insertion [7,65]. The preformed shape of customized, 3D-printed molar shells thus obviates the need to adapt bands, which may increase comfort for both the patient and practitioner [7,40]. Even though limited evidence is available, the digitally printed shells seem to provide clinically acceptable survival rates [7].

5.2. Computer-Aided Manufactured Mentoplates

Conventional *Mentoplates* were shown to be effective, especially in case of maxillary protraction in early class III treatments [28,29]. Using computer-aided manufacturing, *Mentoplates* can be designed to hold supra-constructions with various functional elements of high precision, including sliding mechanics for distalization or mesialization of posterior teeth, which increase the range of treatment options (Figure 9).

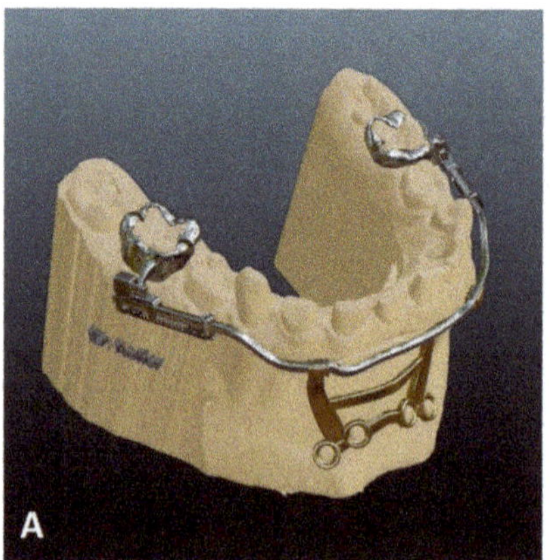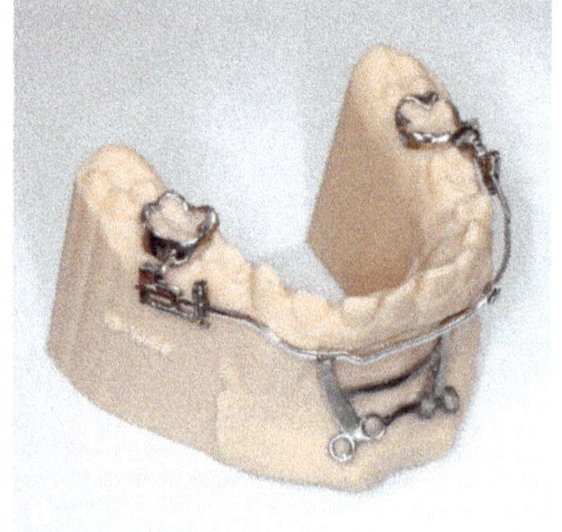

Figure 9. 3D-printed *Mentoplate* with mesial-slider supra-construction: (**A**) Digital design. (**B**) Finished printed appliance (software: Blender, Blender Foundation).

Both conventional and digitally manufactured appliances with a submucosal extent can be made from titanium alloys. Under local anesthesia or narcosis, the oral surgeon prepares a mucoperiosteal flap, revealing the bone structures of the chin. Conventional *Mentoplates* are adapted by bending them manually to fit the chin bone. The two extension arms are shortened and formed either straight or bent into a hook. Depending on the purpose of the treatment, they should penetrate the soft tissue at the mucogingival border or within the attached mucosa to avoid infection and eventually loss of the appliance.

3D-printed appliances do not require adaptation within surgery as they are already customized regarding the individual anatomical situation. While guides for palatal appliances lead the drill during the implants' insertion, osteosynthesis screws are directly applied into their connectors. Therefore, the guide must stabilize the *Mentoplate* in the correct position while the screws are inserted. For this purpose, it proved efficient to assemble the *Mentoplate* with its supra-construction and employ the posterior shells as orientation. To achieve stable triangular support, a printed guide can be mounted onto the lower incisors as well as on the supra-construction, ensuring vertical control (Figure 10). After fastening the screws, the guide can be removed, and the active elements can be adjusted as indicated. After the screws are applied, the flap can be adapted and sutured.

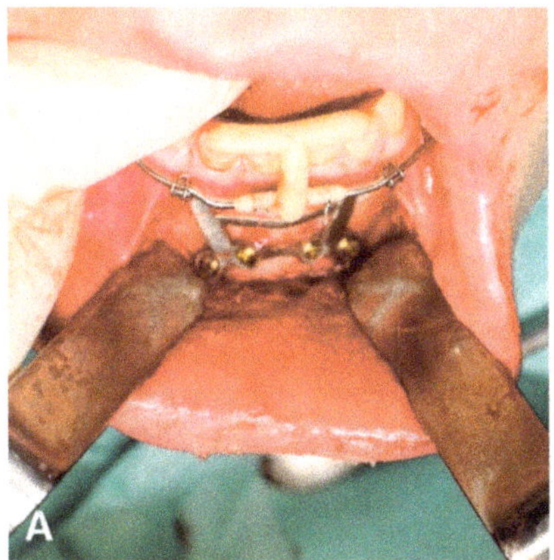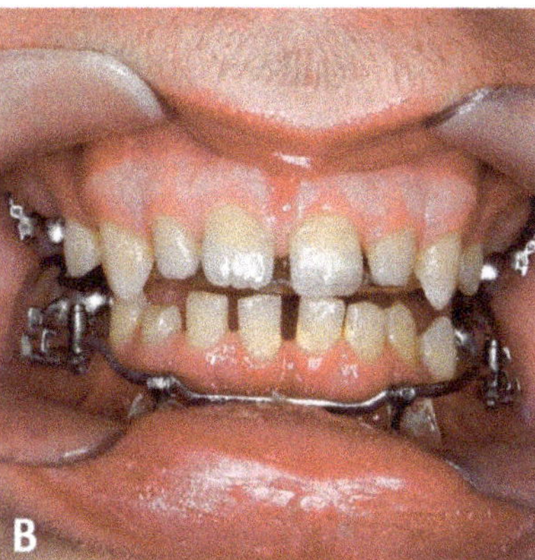

Figure 10. Clinical installation of a CAD/CAM manufactured *Mentoplate* with mesial-slider supra-construction. (**A**) Surgical insertion and anterior vertical control with guide. (**B**) Intraoral situation with installed appliance.

6. Conclusions

The incorporation of a digital workflow with computer-aided design enabled fabrication of customized 3D-printed metal orthodontic appliances. In complex cases requiring additional anchorage, the incorporation of skeletal anchorage may increase the spectrum of treatment options and enable highly time-efficient treatments with increased patient comfort. Nonetheless, digital workflows necessitate an initial training period and may be associated with high acquisition costs, especially when applied in-house. As errors during the process can accumulate from the different steps, accurate planning and validation of a proper fit prior to insertion of screws and appliances is strongly recommended.

Author Contributions: Conceptualization, M.K. and K.B.; software, D.D.; investigation, M.K. and K.B.; resources, D.D.; writing—original draft preparation, M.K.; writing—review and editing, M.K., D.D. and K.B.; visualization, M.K. and K.B.; supervision, M.K., D.D. and K.B.; project administration, M.K., D.D. and K.B. All authors have read and agreed to the published version of the manuscript.

Funding: This research received no external funding.

Informed Consent Statement: Written informed consent has been obtained from the patients to publish this paper.

Data Availability Statement: Not applicable.

Conflicts of Interest: The authors declare no conflict of interest.

References

1. Wong, K.C. 3D-printed patient-specific applications in orthopedics. *Orthop. Res. Rev.* **2016**, *8*, 57–66. [CrossRef] [PubMed]
2. Tack, P.; Victor, J.; Gemmel, P.; Annemans, L. 3D-printing techniques in a medical setting: A systematic literature review. *Biomed. Eng. Online* **2016**, *15*, 115. [CrossRef] [PubMed]
3. Bauermeister, A.J.; Zuriarrain, A.; Newman, M.I. Three-Dimensional Printing in Plastic and Reconstructive Surgery: A Systematic Review. *Ann. Plast. Surg.* **2016**, *77*, 569–576. [CrossRef] [PubMed]
4. Jamróz, W.; Szafraniec, J.; Kurek, M.; Jachowicz, R. 3D Printing in Pharmaceutical and Medical Applications—Recent Achievements and Challenges. *Pharm. Res.* **2018**, *35*, 176. [CrossRef] [PubMed]
5. Della Bona, A.; Cantelli, V.; Britto, V.T.; Collares, K.F.; Stansbury, J.W. 3D printing restorative materials using a stereolithographic technique: A systematic review. *Dent. Mater.* **2021**, *37*, 336–350. [CrossRef]
6. Tian, Y.; Chen, C.; Xu, X.; Wang, J.; Hou, X.; Li, K.; Lu, X.; Shi, H.; Lee, E.S.; Jiang, H.B. A Review of 3D Printing in Dentistry: Technologies, Affecting Factors, and Applications. *Scanning* **2021**, *2021*, 9950131. [CrossRef]
7. Graf, S.; Cornelis, M.A.; Hauber Gameiro, G.; Cattaneo, P.M. Computer-aided design and manufacture of hyrax devices: Can we really go digital? *Am. J. Orthod. Dentofac. Orthop.* **2017**, *152*, 870–874. [CrossRef]

8.   Graf, S.; Vasudavan, S.; Wilmes, B. CAD-CAM design and 3-dimensional printing of mini-implant retained orthodontic appliances. *Am. J. Orthod. Dentofac. Orthop.* **2018**, *154*, 877–882. [CrossRef]

9.   Clemente, R.; Contardo, L.; Greco, C.; Di Lenarda, R.; Perinetti, G. Class III Treatment with Skeletal and Dental Anchorage: A Review of Comparative Effects. *BioMed Res. Int.* **2018**, *2018*, 7946019. [CrossRef]

10. Wilmes, B.; Olthoff, G.; Drescher, D. Comparison of skeletal and conventional anchorage methods in conjunction with pre-operative decompensation of a skeletal class III malocclusion. *J. Orofac. Orthop.* **2009**, *70*, 297–305. [CrossRef]

11. Proffit, W.R.; Fields, H.W. *Contemporary Orthodontics*; Mosby-Year Book: St. Louis, MO, USA, 1993.

12. Nienkemper, M.; Wilmes, B.; Lübberink, G.; Ludwig, B.; Drescher, D. Extrusion of impacted teeth using mini-implant mechanics. *J. Clin. Orthod.* **2012**, *46*, 150–155, quiz 183. [PubMed]

13. Nienkemper, M.; Handschel, J.; Drescher, D. Systematic review of mini-implant displacement under orthodontic loading. *Int. J. Oral Sci.* **2014**, *6*, 1–6. [CrossRef] [PubMed]

14. Wilmes, B.; Willmann, J.; Stocker, B.; Drescher, D. Mini-Implantate zur kieferorthopädischen Verankerung im anterioren Gaumen, mediane vs. paramediane Insertion. *Inf. Orthod. Kieferorthopädie* **2015**, *47*, 243–248. [CrossRef]

15. Wilmes, B.; Ludwig, B.; Vasudavan, S.; Nienkemper, M.; Drescher, D. The T-Zone: Median vs. Paramedian Insertion of Palatal Mini-Implants. *J. Clin. Orthod.* **2016**, *50*, 543–551.

16. Becker, K.; Pliska, A.; Busch, C.; Wilmes, B.; Wolf, M.; Drescher, D. Efficacy of orthodontic mini implants for en masse retraction in the maxilla: A systematic review and meta-analysis. *Int. J. Implant. Dent.* **2018**, *4*, 35. [CrossRef] [PubMed]

17. Becker, K.; Wilmes, B.; Grandjean, C.; Vasudavan, S.; Drescher, D. Skeletally anchored mesialization of molars using digitized casts and two surface-matching approaches: Analysis of treatment effects. *J. Orofac. Orthop.* **2018**, *79*, 11–18. [CrossRef]

18. Fritz, U.; Ehmer, A.; Diedrich, P. Clinical suitability of titanium microscrews for orthodontic anchorage-preliminary experiences. *J. Orofac. Orthop.* **2004**, *65*, 410–418. [CrossRef]

19. Wilmes, B.; Drescher, D. A miniscrew system with interchangeable abutments. *J. Clin. Orthod.* **2008**, *42*, 574–580.

20. Ludwig, B.; Glasl, B.; Bowman, S.J.; Wilmes, B.; Kinzinger, G.S.M.; Lisson, J.A. Anatomical guidelines for miniscrew insertion: Palatal sites. *J. Clin. Orthod.* **2011**, *45*, 433–441.

21. Mohammed, H.; Wafaie, K.; Rizk, M.Z.; Almuzian, M.; Sosly, R.; Bearn, D.R. Role of anatomical sites and correlated risk factors on the survival of orthodontic miniscrew implants: A systematic review and meta-analysis. *Prog. Orthod.* **2018**, *19*, 36. [CrossRef]

22. Nienkemper, M.; Pauls, A.; Ludwig, B.; Wilmes, B.; Drescher, D. Preprosthetic molar uprighting using skeletal anchorage. *J. Clin. Orthod.* **2013**, *47*, 433–437. [PubMed]

23. Ludwig, B.; Glasl, B.; Kinzinger, G.S.M.; Lietz, T.; Lisson, J.A. Anatomical guidelines for miniscrew insertion: Vestibular interradicular sites. *J. Clin. Orthod.* **2011**, *45*, 165–173.

24. Poggio, P.M.; Incorvati, C.; Velo, S.; Carano, A. "Safe zones": A guide for miniscrew positioning in the maxillary and mandibular arch. *Angle Orthod.* **2006**, *76*, 191–197.

25. Chen, Y.H.; Chang, H.H.; Chen, Y.J.; Lee, D.; Chiang, H.H.; Yao, C.C. Root contact during insertion of miniscrews for orthodontic anchorage increases the failure rate: An animal study. *Clin. Oral Implant. Res.* **2008**, *19*, 99–106. [CrossRef] [PubMed]

26. Kadioglu, O.; Büyükyilmaz, T.; Zachrisson, B.U.; Maino, B.G. Contact damage to root surfaces of premolars touching miniscrews during orthodontic treatment. *Am. J. Orthod. Dentofac. Orthop.* **2008**, *134*, 353–360. [CrossRef]

27. Arqub, S.A.; Gandhi, V.; Mehta, S.; Palo, L.; Upadhyay, M.; Yadav, S. Survival estimates and risk factors for failure of palatal and buccal mini-implants. *Angle Orthod.* **2021**, *91*, 756–763. [CrossRef]

28. Wilmes, B.; Nienkemper, M.; Ludwig, B.; Kau, C.H.; Drescher, D. Early Class III treatment with a hybrid hyrax-mentoplate combination. *J. Clin. Orthod.* **2011**, *45*, 15–21.

29. Katyal, V.; Wilmes, B.; Nienkemper, M.; Darendeliler, M.A.; Sampson, W.; Drescher, D. The efficacy of Hybrid Hyrax-Mentoplate combination in early Class III treatment: A novel approach and pilot study. *Aust. Orthod. J.* **2016**, *32*, 88–96. [CrossRef]

30. Freudenthaler, J.W.; Haas, R.; Bantleon, H.P. Bicortical titanium screws for critical orthodontic anchorage in the mandible: A preliminary report on clinical applications. *Clin. Oral Implants Res.* **2001**, *12*, 358–363. [CrossRef]

31. Nienkemper, M.; Pauls, A.; Ludwig, B.; Wilmes, B.; Drescher, D. Multifunctional use of palatal mini-implants. *J. Clin. Orthod.* **2012**, *46*, 679–686.

32. Becker, K.; de Gabriele, R.; Dallatana, G.; Trelenberg-Stoll, V.; Wilmes, B.; Drescher, D. *3-D-Planung für Implantate in der Kieferorthopädie*; Quintessence Publishing: Berlin, Germany, 2018; pp. 147–154.

33. Willmann, J.; Wilmes, B.; Becker, K.; Drescher, D. Hybrid Hyrax Direct. *Kieferorthopädie* **2020**, *34*, 249–257.

34. Isidor, F. Histological evaluation of peri-implant bone at implants subjected to occlusal overload or plaque accumulation. *Clin. Oral Implants Res.* **1997**, *8*, 1–9. [CrossRef] [PubMed]

35. Isidor, F. Loss of osseointegration caused by occlusal load of oral implants. A clinical and radiographic study in monkeys. *Clin. Oral Implants Res.* **1996**, *7*, 143–152. [CrossRef] [PubMed]

36. Jedliński, M.; Mazur, M.; Grocholewicz, K.; Janiszewska-Olszowska, J. 3D Scanners in Orthodontics-Current Knowledge and Future Perspectives—A Systematic Review. *Int. J. Environ. Res. Public Health* **2021**, *18*, 1121. [CrossRef]

37. Aragón, M.L.; Pontes, L.F.; Bichara, L.M.; Flores-Mir, C.; Normando, D. Validity and reliability of intraoral scanners compared to conventional gypsum models measurements: A systematic review. *Eur. J. Orthod.* **2016**, *38*, 429–434. [CrossRef] [PubMed]

38. Glisic, O.; Hoejbjerre, L.; Sonnesen, L. A comparison of patient experience, chair-side time, accuracy of dental arch measurements and costs of acquisition of dental models. *Angle Orthod.* **2019**, *89*, 868–875. [CrossRef]

39. Groth, C.; Kravitz, N.D.; Jones, P.E.; Graham, J.W.; Redmond, W.R. Three-dimensional printing technology. *J. Clin. Orthod.* **2014**, *48*, 475–485.
40. Willmann, J.H.; Wilmes, B.; Chhatwani, S.; Drescher, D. Klinische Anwendung des digitalen Workflows am Beispiel von Mini-Implantaten. *Inf. Orthod. Kieferorthopädie* **2020**, *52*, 121–127. [CrossRef]
41. Möhlhenrich, S.C.; Brandt, M.; Kniha, K.; Bock, A.; Prescher, A.; Hölzle, F.; Modabber, A.; Danesh, G. Suitability of virtual plaster models superimposed with the lateral cephalogram for guided paramedian orthodontic mini-implant placement with regard to the bone support. *J. Orofac. Orthop.* **2020**, *81*, 340–349. [CrossRef]
42. Kniha, K.; Brandt, M.; Bock, A.; Modabber, A.; Prescher, A.; Hölzle, F.; Danesh, G.; Möhlhenrich, S.C. Accuracy of fully guided orthodontic mini-implant placement evaluated by cone-beam computed tomography: A study involving human cadaver heads. *Clin. Oral Investig.* **2021**, *25*, 1299–1306. [CrossRef]
43. Gabriele, O.; Dallatana, G.; Riva, R.; Vasudavan, S.; Wilmes, B. The easy driver for placement of palatal mini-implants and a maxillary expander in a single appointment. *J. Clin. Orthod. JCO* **2017**, *51*, 728–737. [PubMed]
44. Petzold, R.; Zeilhofer, H.F.; Kalender, W.A. Rapid protyping technology in medicine-basics and applications. *Comput. Med. Imaging Graph.* **1999**, *23*, 277–284. [CrossRef]
45. Möhlhenrich, S.C.; Brandt, M.; Kniha, K.; Prescher, A.; Hölzle, F.; Modabber, A.; Wolf, M.; Peters, F. Accuracy of orthodontic mini-implants placed at the anterior palate by tooth-borne or gingiva-borne guide support: A cadaveric study. *Clin. Oral Investig.* **2019**, *23*, 4425–4431. [CrossRef] [PubMed]
46. Jung, B.A.; Wehrbein, H.; Heuser, L.; Kunkel, M. Vertical palatal bone dimensions on lateral cephalometry and cone-beam computed tomography: Implications for palatal implant placement. *Clin. Oral Implants Res.* **2011**, *22*, 664–668. [CrossRef] [PubMed]
47. Graf, S.; Tarraf, N.E.; Kravitz, N.D. Three-dimensional metal printed orthodontic laboratory appliances. *Semin. Orthod.* **2021**, *27*, 189–193. [CrossRef]
48. Mazzoli, A. Selective laser sintering in biomedical engineering. *Med. Biol. Eng. Comput.* **2013**, *51*, 245–256. [CrossRef]
49. Mazzoli, A.; Germani, M.; Moriconi, G. Application of optical digitizing techniques to evaluate the shape accuracy of anatomical models derived from computed tomography data. *J. Oral Maxillofac. Surg.* **2007**, *65*, 1410–1418. [CrossRef]
50. Gokuldoss, P.K.; Kolla, S.; Eckert, J. Additive Manufacturing Processes: Selective Laser Melting, Electron Beam Melting and Binder Jetting-Selection Guidelines. *Materials* **2017**, *10*, 672. [CrossRef]
51. Al Maaz, A.; Thompson, G.A.; Drago, C.; An, H.; Berzins, D. Effect of finish line design and metal alloy on the marginal and internal gaps of selective laser melting printed copings. *J. Prosthet. Dent.* **2019**, *122*, 143–151. [CrossRef]
52. Presotto, A.G.C.; Barão, V.A.R.; Bhering, C.L.B.; Mesquita, M.F. Dimensional precision of implant-supported frameworks fabricated by 3D printing. *J. Prosthet. Dent.* **2019**, *122*, 38–45. [CrossRef]
53. Akçin, E.T.; Güncü, M.B.; Aktaş, G.; Aslan, Y. Effect of manufacturing techniques on the marginal and internal fit of cobalt-chromium implant-supported multiunit frameworks. *J. Prosthet. Dent.* **2018**, *120*, 715–720. [CrossRef] [PubMed]
54. Bae, S.; Hong, M.H.; Lee, H.; Lee, C.H.; Hong, M.; Lee, J.; Lee, D.H. Reliability of Metal 3D Printing with Respect to the Marginal Fit of Fixed Dental Prostheses: A Systematic Review and Meta-Analysis. *Materials* **2020**, *13*, 4781. [CrossRef] [PubMed]
55. Lin, L.; Fang, Y.; Liao, Y.; Chen, G.; Gao, C.; Zhu, P. 3D printing and digital processing techniques in dentistry: A review of literature. *Adv. Eng. Mater.* **2019**, *21*, 1801013. [CrossRef]
56. Tipnis, N.P.; Burgess, D.J. Sterilization of implantable polymer-based medical devices: A review. *Int. J. Pharm.* **2018**, *544*, 455–460. [CrossRef]
57. Jeremy, W.; Thampi, R.; Marc, L.; Michael, K.; Quan, N. Sterilization of bedside 3D-printed devices for use in the operating room. *Ann. 3D Print. Med.* **2022**, *5*, 100045.
58. Ghobeira, R.; Philips, C.; Declercq, H.; Cools, P.; De Geyter, N.; Cornelissen, R.; Morent, R. Effects of different sterilization methods on the physico-chemical and bioresponsive properties of plasma-treated polycaprolactone films. *Biomed. Mater.* **2017**, *12*, 015017. [CrossRef]
59. Sharma, N.; Cao, S.; Msallem, B.; Kunz, C.; Brantner, P.; Honigmann, P.; Thieringer, F.M. Effects of Steam Sterilization on 3D Printed Biocompatible Resin Materials for Surgical Guides-An Accuracy Assessment Study. *J. Clin. Med.* **2020**, *9*, 1506. [CrossRef]
60. Toro, M.; Cardona, A.; Restrepo, D.; Buitrago, L. Does vaporized hydrogen peroxide sterilization affect the geometrical properties of anatomic models and guides 3D printed from computed tomography images? *3D Print Med.* **2021**, *7*, 29. [CrossRef]
61. Pérez Davila, S.; González Rodríguez, L.; Chiussi, S.; Serra, J.; González, P. How to Sterilize Polylactic Acid Based Medical Devices? *Polymers* **2021**, *13*, 2115. [CrossRef]
62. Melsen, B.; Costa, A. Immediate loading of implants used for orthodontic anchorage. *Clin. Orthod. Res.* **2000**, *3*, 23–28. [CrossRef]
63. Rismanchian, M.; Raji, S.H.; Razavi, S.M.; Rick, D.T.; Davoudi, A. Application of Orthodontic Immediate Force on Dental Implants: Histomorphologic and Histomorphometric Assessment. *Ann. Maxillofac. Surg.* **2017**, *7*, 11–17. [PubMed]
64. Rossini, G.; Parrini, S.; Castroflorio, T.; Deregibus, A.; Debernardi, C.L. Diagnostic accuracy and measurement sensitivity of digital models for orthodontic purposes: A systematic review. *Am. J. Orthod. Dentofac. Orthop.* **2016**, *149*, 161–170. [CrossRef] [PubMed]
65. Shannon, T.; Groth, C. Be your own manufacturer: 3D printing intraoral appliances. In *Seminars in Orthodontics Seminars*; WB Saunders: Philadelphia, PA, USA, 2021.

applied sciences

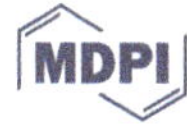

Article

Impact of Steam Autoclaving on the Mechanical Properties of 3D-Printed Resins Used for Insertion Guides in Orthodontics and Implant Dentistry

Anna Kirschner [1], Samuel David [1], Giulia Brunello [2,3], Ludger Keilig [4], Dieter Drescher [1], Christoph Bourauel [4] and Kathrin Becker [1,*]

[1] Department of Orthodontics, University of Dusseldorf, 40225 Dusseldorf, Germany; anna.kirschner@uni-duesseldorf.de (A.K.); samuel.david@uni-duesseldorf.de (S.D.); drescher@med.uni-duesseldorf.de (D.D.)

[2] Department of Oral Surgery, University of Dusseldorf, 40225 Dusseldorf, Germany; giulia.brunello@med.uni-duesseldorf.de

[3] Department of Neurosciences, University of Padua, 35128 Padua, Italy

[4] Oral Technology, University of Bonn, 53111 Bonn, Germany; ludger.keilig@uni-bonn.de (L.K.); bourauel@uni-bonn.de (C.B.)

* Correspondence: kathrin.becker@med.uni-duesseldorf.de; Tel.: +49-211-811-8145

Abstract: Guided implant placement has been shown to be more accurate than free-handed insertion. Still, implant position deviations occur and could possibly pose risks. Thus, there is a quest to identify factors that might impair the accuracy of implantation protocols using templates. This study aimed to investigate the influence of autoclaving cycles (cycle 1: 121 °C, 1 bar, 20.5 min; cycle 2: 134 °C, 2 bar, 5.5 min) on the Vickers hardness and flexural modulus of five different materials used for 3D-printed insertion guides. The specimens were subjected to Vickers hardness tests, showing significant changes in the Vickers hardness for two and three materials out of five for cycle 1 and 2, respectively. The results of the three-point bending tests (n = 15 specimens per material) showed decreasing flexural moduli after autoclaving. However, changes were significant only for one material, which presented a significant decrease in the flexural modulus after cycle 2. No significant changes were detected after cycle 1. In conclusion, our findings show that autoclaving can alter the mechanical properties of the templates to some extent, especially with cycle 2. Whether these modifications are associated with dimensional changes of the templates and reduced accuracy of the implantation protocols remains to be investigated.

Keywords: flexural modulus; hardness; surgical template; sterilization; additive manufacturing

Citation: Kirschner, A.; David, S.; Brunello, G.; Keilig, L.; Drescher, D.; Bourauel, C.; Becker, K. Impact of Steam Autoclaving on the Mechanical Properties of 3D-Printed Resins Used for Insertion Guides in Orthodontics and Implant Dentistry. *Appl. Sci.* **2022**, *12*, 6195. https://doi.org/10.3390/app12126195

Academic Editor: Anthony William Coleman

Received: 30 May 2022
Accepted: 15 June 2022
Published: 17 June 2022

Publisher's Note: MDPI stays neutral with regard to jurisdictional claims in published maps and institutional affiliations.

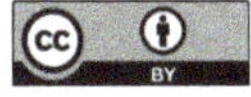

1. Introduction

In recent years, computer-guided surgery in combination with digital backward-planning gained popularity among clinicians in the field of implant dentistry and also in orthodontics for mini-implant placement. Especially in challenging situations, accurate transfer of the virtually planned position of the implants may increase the safety of the intervention, and improve patient comfort as a consequence of reduced operation time and invasiveness [1]. Guided implant surgery using surgical templates was found to be more accurate compared to free-handed implant placement, exhibiting significantly lower angular, coronal, and apical deviations between the intended and the actual implant positions [2,3].

Despite these benefits, a mean coronal deviation of 1.3 mm (95% CI: 1.09 mm; 1.56 mm) with values up to 2.2 mm and a mean apical deviation of 1.5 mm (95% CI: 1.29 mm; 1.62 mm) with values up to 2.5 mm have been reported for computer-guided implant insertion [4]. These distances should be incorporated into the virtual planning to reduce the risk of permanent damage to adjacent anatomical structures. Nevertheless, this risk cannot be fully eliminated and a safe distance between the implants and the anatomical structures should be considered in the planning phase [5]. These circumstances stress the importance of investigating factors that could provoke the loss of accuracy, so that the risk–benefit ratio of computer-guided implantation protocols can be optimized in the future. As stated in the EU Medical Devices Regulation (MDR), it is crucial to minimize all the "known and foreseeable risks and any undesirable side-effects" and weigh them against possible benefits of the chosen protocol [6].

Formerly identified factors influencing the accuracy of guided implantation include the support of the surgical template, favoring tooth- and mucosa-supported surgical templates over bone-supported ones [7]. In the case of mucosa-supported surgical templates, the mucosal thickness at the insertion site was found to affect implant placement accuracy, whereby increased tissue thickness seems to lower the accuracy and may require flap preparation for more accurate results [8,9]. Furthermore, the quality of radiographic image data and the usage of intraoral scanning devices might have an impact on the accuracy of guided implantation protocols [10–13]. In addition, the fit and the length of the metallic drilling sleeves embedded within the surgical template and the drilling distance could determine the extent of implant position deviations [14,15].

Surgical guides have been widely employed in implant dentistry. Recently, mini-implant insertion templates were introduced in orthodontics to increase the safety and accuracy of the procedure [16]. Few studies confirmed an increased accuracy following guided placement of orthodontic implants [17]. In the anterior palate, insertion templates not only favor ideal mini-implant positioning in accordance with the variable bone height available [18], but also facilitate simultaneous placement of skeletally anchored orthodontic appliances in a digital workflow [19].

Nowadays, guides are usually produced in resin-based materials using additive manufacturing technologies [20]. Recent studies have suggested that the influence of different 3D-printers on the accuracy of the protocol is negligible [21,22], whereas dimensional changes caused by prolonged storage have been reported [23]. Another critical aspect that might alter the accuracy of implant insertion and that has not gained much attention so far is the impact of steam autoclaving. The sterilization of the templates is fundamental, as they can come temporarily in contact with blood. According to international hygiene guidelines, including the Center for Disease Control and Prevention (CDC, USA) and the EU Regulations, they are critical medical devices and have to be sterilized before usage [6,24]. Few recent studies could not find significant changes in template dimension after autoclaving [25–27], whereas the impact on biomechanical properties remains unclear. Alteration of the biomechanical properties, such as flexural properties and hardness of the template materials, might lead to inaccuracies in implant insertion. Thus, there is a quest for studies assessing the influence of steam autoclaving parameters, such as temperature, pressure, and duration of autoclaving. Furthermore, the effect of autoclaving on different resin-based materials manufactured with different printing methods, such as stereolithography (SLA), liquid crystal display stereolithography (LCD-SLA), and digital light processing (DLP), remains to be clarified.

Therefore, the aim of this study was to evaluate the influence of steam autoclaving parameters on the Vickers hardness and flexural modulus of 3D-printed resin-based templates, manufactured using different resin materials and printing methods. The null hypotheses were that being subjected to autoclaving did not significantly change the specimen Vickers hardness HV 0.5 and the flexural modulus.

2. Materials and Methods

2.1. 3D-Printed Specimens Preparation

As the test standard DIN EN ISO 178 requires the usage of test pieces with a length (l) height (h) ratio of l/h = 20 for 3-point bending tests on polymer materials, a virtual model of the specimens with the dimensions 2 mm × 25 mm × 40 mm was designed using the software 3D-Builder (Microsoft, Redmond, WA, USA). In total, 75 specimens (i.e., 15 for each of the 5 materials) were printed for 3-point bending tests and Vickers hardness tests. With regard to test groups, two different digital light processing (DLP) printers (group 1: NextDent 5100, Vertex-Dental B.V., Soesteberg, The Netherlands; group 2: ASIGA MAX, Pluradent GmbH & Co. KG, Offenbach, Germany), one desktop stereolithography (SLA) printer (group 3: Form 3, Formlabs Inc., Sommerville, MA, USA), and one liquid crystal display stereolithography (LCD-SLA) printer (group 4: Slash Plus, UniZ Technology LLC., San Diego, CA, USA) were used. The samples were produced using four different 3D printing resins, one for each printing machine (group 1: NextDent SG, Vertex-Dental B.V.; group 2: Optiprint Guide, dentona AG, Dortmund, Germany; group 3: Dental SG, Formlabs Inc.; group 4: zSG Amber, UniZ Technology LLC.). All of the resins mentioned before are authorized by the manufacturer for steam autoclaving and printing with the particular printer utilized. The resin used in group 0 (E-Guide, Envisiontec Inc., Dearborn, MI, USA) is not authorized by the manufacturer for steam autoclaving, but only for immersion disinfection. It was printed with the DLP printer authorized by the manufacturer (Micro Plus XL, Envisiontec Inc.).

All specimens were printed such that the printing layers were parallel to the longer edge and perpendicular to the support structures and to the shorter edges, as recommended by Quintana et al. [28].

Five specimens per group (total n = 25) were not subjected to autoclaving and were used as controls. Ten specimens per group were sterilized by two different vacuum steam autoclaving programs (Vacuklav 44-B, MELAG oHG, Berlin, Germany): 5 specimens at 121 °C, 1 bar, and 20.5 min (cycle 1), while the remaining 5 were sterilized at 134 °C, 2 bar, and 5.5 min (cycle 2). A summary is provided in Table 1.

Table 1. Printers and resins used in this study, with details of the number of specimens per group and subgroup.

Group [§]	Printing Method	Printer, Manufacturer	Resin, Manufacturer
0	DLP	Micro Plus XL, Envisiontec Inc.	E-Guide, Envisiontec Inc.
1	DLP	NextDent 5100, Vertex-Dental B.V.	NextDent SG, Vertex-Dental B.V.
2	DLP	ASIGA MAX, Pluradent GmbH & Co. KG	Optiprint Guide, dentona AG
3	SLA	Form 3, Formlabs Inc.	Dental SG, Formlabs Inc.
4	LCD-SLA	Slash Plus, UniZ Technology LLC.	zSG Amber, UniZ Technology LLC.

[§] for each of the five groups, 15 samples divided in 3 subgroups (n = 5 per subgroup): untreated; cycle 1 (121 °C, 1 bar, 20.5 min); cycle 2 (134 °C, 2 bar, 5.5 min). DLP: digital light processing; LCD-SLA: liquid crystal display stereolithography; SLA: stereolithography.

2.2. Mechanical Tests

The Vickers hardness test was performed on three specimens of each subgroup using the hardness testing machine ZHV20/Z2.5 (Zwick-Roell GmbH & Co. KG, Ulm, Germany) and repeated 5 times. Tests were run according to the ISO/TS 19278 norm. A 136° pyramidal indenter was pressed into the material with a force (F) of 4.903 N for 10 s. Images of the resulting impression were acquired using the optical microscope with a magnification of 20:1, that the hardness testing machine ZHV20/Z2.5 is equipped with. The diagonals d_1 and d_2 of the impression were measured manually using the software testXpert (Zwick-Roell GmbH & Co. KG) (Figure 1). Then, the average diagonal d and Vickers hardness HV0.5 were calculated using the following equations.

$$d = (d_1 + d_2)/2 \tag{1}$$

$$HV0.5 = 0.1891 \times F/d^2 \tag{2}$$

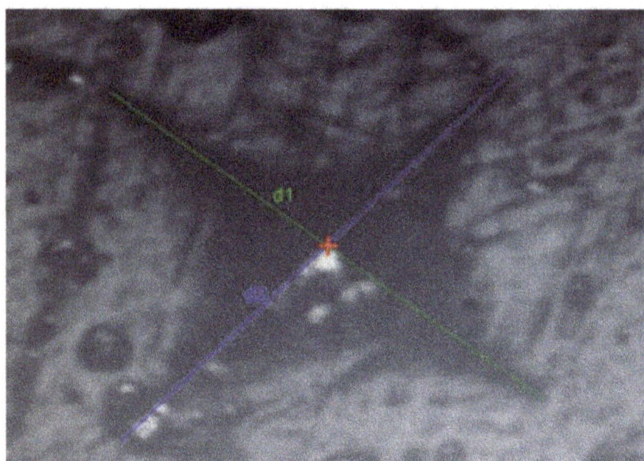

Figure 1. Microscopic image of the impression left by the pyramidal indenter during the Vickers hardness test with markings of diagonals d_1 and d_2.

To evaluate autoclaving-induced changes in terms of flexural properties of the tested materials, a 3-point bending test was performed following the test standard DIN EN ISO 178 on all specimens ($n = 75$). The tests were performed using the material testing machine ZMART.PRO (Zwick-Roell GmbH & Co. KG) with a testing stamp radius of 5 mm that bends the specimens with a speed of 2 mm/s. The specimens were positioned such that the acquired ratio of the test piece length (l) to the distance between the support points (d) was l/d = 16 (Figure 2). The software testXpert (Zwick-Roell GmbH & Co. KG) was used to detect the flexural moduli.

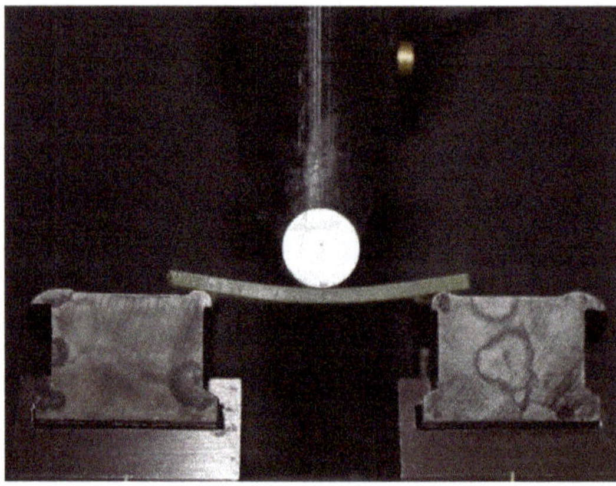

Figure 2. 3-point bending test of a specimen from group 3.

2.3. Statistical Analysis

The statistical analysis was performed using Excel 2016 (Microsoft). A convenience sample size was determined, based on similar publications in this field [29,30]. For Vickers hardness, repeated measurements on the same specimen were pooled. For each resin/printer combination and autoclaving protocol, the mean ± standard deviation (M ± SD) Vickers hardness and flexural modulus were calculated. The Shapiro–Wilk test was used to assess whether measured data were normally distributed. The normal distribution of residues was validated through Q-Q plots. Homoscedasticity was verified by conducting a Levene test.

The ANOVA and post hoc *t*-test with Bonferroni correction were used to assess differences among autoclaving protocols for each printer/resin combination. If the assumptions for ANOVA were not met, a Kruskal–Wallis test and a post hoc Bonferroni-corrected Mann–Whitney-U test were utilized instead.

As the measurements of d_1 and d_2 in Vickers hardness testing were performed manually, the reliability of the test method was assessed using the interclass correlation coefficient (ICC), which was calculated based on the 5 repeated measurements.

Results were found significant at $p < 0.05$.

3. Results

3.1. Vickers Hardness

The reliability of the Vickers hardness test ranged from moderate (ICC = 0.58) to excellent (ICC = 0.99). The mean Vickers hardness (in HV0.5) and standard deviations ranged from 13.50 ± 2.62 to 29.16 ± 6.83 for the untreated subgroups. After the specimens were autoclaved with cycle 1, the Vickers hardness ranged from 6.94 ± 2.21 to 27.67 ± 5.42. After being subjected to cycle 2, the Vickers hardness ranged from 10.52 ± 1.05 to 25.30 ± 1.65.

The results of the Vickers hardness test are given in Table 2, and corresponding boxplots are provided in Figure 3. In three out of five resin/printer groups, the Kruskal–Wallis test pointed at qualitative differences (group 0, group 2, and group 3). In these groups, a post hoc test was conducted. In group 0, the Vickers hardness of the specimens autoclaved with cycle 1 significantly decreased and almost halved compared to the untreated control ($p < 0.001$), whereas cycle 2 yielded significantly higher Vickers hardness values ($p < 0.001$. In group 2, the Vickers hardness of cycle 1 increased slightly ($p = 0.359$) compared to the untreated control, whereas the Vickers hardness of the cycle 2 subgroup was significantly lower compared to the untreated control and cycle 1 groups ($p < 0.001$, respectively). In group 3, a higher Vickers hardness was found for both autoclaving protocols (untreated vs. cycle 1: $p = 0.010$; untreated vs. cycle 2: $p < 0.001$), whereas no significant differences were found between the two autoclaving cycles.

Table 2. Results of the Vickers hardness test and statistical analysis.

Group [§]	ICC	Subgroup [§§]	Vickers Hardness [HV0.5] M ± SD	Kruskal–Wallis H (2)	p_H	Comparison	U	z	p_U	r
0	0.993	untreated	13.50 ± 2.62	35.896	<0.001 ***	untreated vs. cycle 1	8	−4.334	<0.001 ***	−0.791
		cycle 1	6.94 ± 2.21			untreated vs. cycle 2	9	−4.293	<0.001 ***	−0.784
		cycle 2	19.57 ± 2.04			cycle 1 vs. cycle 2	1	−4.625	<0.001 ***	−0.844
1	0.582	untreated	29.16 ± 6.83	5.847	0.054	-	-	-	-	-
		cycle 1	27.67 ± 5.42			-	-	-	-	-
		cycle 2	25.30 ± 1.65			-	-	-	-	-
2	0.945	untreated	14.14 ± 2.33	26.303	<0.001 ***	untreated vs. cycle 1	75	−1.555	0.359	−0.284
		cycle 1	16.00 ± 3.06			untreated vs. cycle 2	26	−3.588	0.001 **	−0.655
		cycle 2	10.52 ± 1.05			cycle 1 vs. cycle 2	3	−4.542	<0.001 ***	−0.829
3	0.925	untreated	17.12 ± 1.96	22.659	<0.001 ***	untreated vs. cycle 1	42	−2.924	0.010 *	−0.534
		cycle 1	20.80 ± 2.95			untreated vs. cycle 2	1	−4.625	<0.001 ***	−0.844
		cycle 2	23.84 ± 2.24			cycle 1 vs. cycle 2	60	−2.178	0.088	−0.398
4	0.670	untreated	15.67 ± 2.41	1.844	0.398	-	-	-	-	-
		cycle 1	16.96 ± 2.92			-	-	-	-	-
		cycle 2	14.74 ± 1.25			-	-	-	-	-

* $p < 0.05$; ** $p < 0.01$; *** $p < 0.001$; [§] $n = 9$ specimens for each of the 5 groups; [§§] $n = 3$ specimens for each of the 15 subgroups; p_H p-value from Kruskal–Wallis test; p_U p-value from Mann–Whitney-U test.

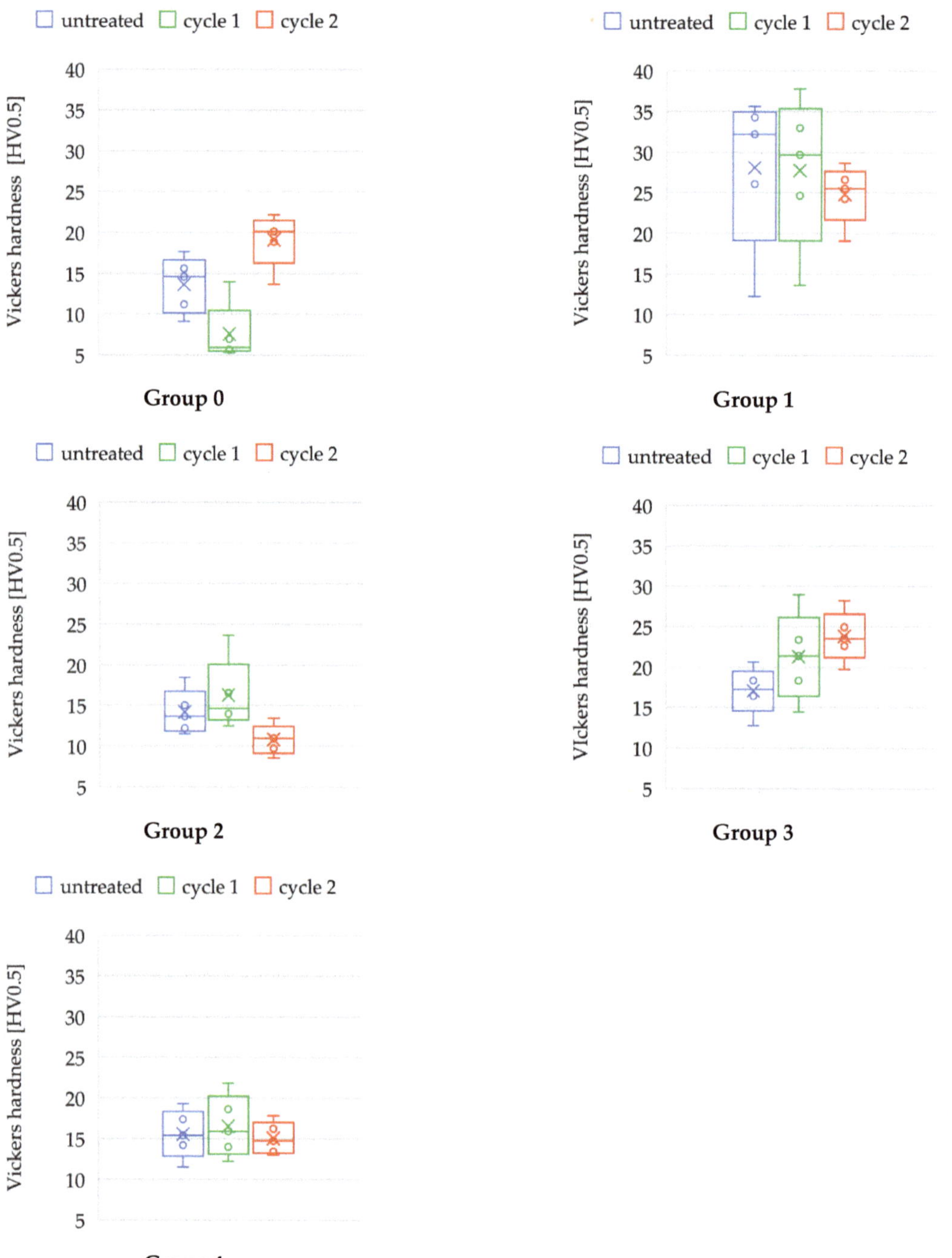

Figure 3. Boxplots: Vickers hardness of the different groups and subgroups. The x represents the mean, the circles represent data points not covered by the boxplots.

3.2. Flexural Modulus

The results of the three-point bending test are summarized in Table 3, and corresponding boxplots are provided in Figure 4. The mean flexural moduli ranged between 1960 MPa and 2762 MPa for the untreated groups. After autoclaving, the mean flexural modulus was lower for each resin/printer combination, ranging from 1205 MPa to 2466 MPa and from 1337 MPa to 2454 MPa for cycles 1 and 2, respectively. However, in the majority of groups, these data failed significance.

Table 3. Results of the three-point bending test and statistical analysis.

Group [§]	Subgroup [§§]	Flexural Modulus E_f [MPa] $M \pm SD$	ANOVA F (2,12)	p_F	Bonferroni-Corrected Post Hoc Test (Students-t, If $p_A < 0.05$) Comparison	t (8)	p_t
0	untreated	1960 ± 405			-	-	-
	cycle 1	1738 ± 494	0.322	0.731	-	-	-
	cycle 2	1812 ± 261			-	-	-
1	untreated	2762 ± 88			untreated vs. cycle 1	2.671	0.085
	cycle 1	2466 ± 203	4.492	0.035 *	untreated vs. cycle 2	3.080	0.045 *
	cycle 2	2454 ± 179			cycle 1 vs. cycle 2	0.089	>0.999
2	untreated	1710 ± 194			-	-	-
	cycle 1	1205 ± 204	1.810	0.206	-	-	-
	cycle 2	1337 ± 613			-	-	-
3	untreated	2280 ± 1108			-	-	-
	cycle 1	2050 ± 542	0.181	0.837	-	-	-
	cycle 2	2372 ± 551			-	-	-
4	untreated	2654 ± 338			-	-	-
	cycle 1	2440 ± 564	0.580	0.575	-	-	-
	cycle 2	2367 ± 536			-	-	-

* $p < 0.05$; [§] $n = 15$ for each of the 5 groups; [§§] $n = 5$ for each of the 15 subgroups; p_F p-value from ANOVA; p_t p-value from Student's t-test.

A qualitative difference was noted in group 1 (ANOVA, $p = 0.035$). The post hoc test revealed a significantly lower flexural modulus following cycle 2 autoclaving compared to the untreated group (t-test, $p = 0.045$). In contrast, no differences were seen following cycle 1 autoclaving compared to the untreated control (t-test, $p = 0.085$). However, there were no significant differences in flexural modulus between the two autoclaving protocols ($p > 0.999$).

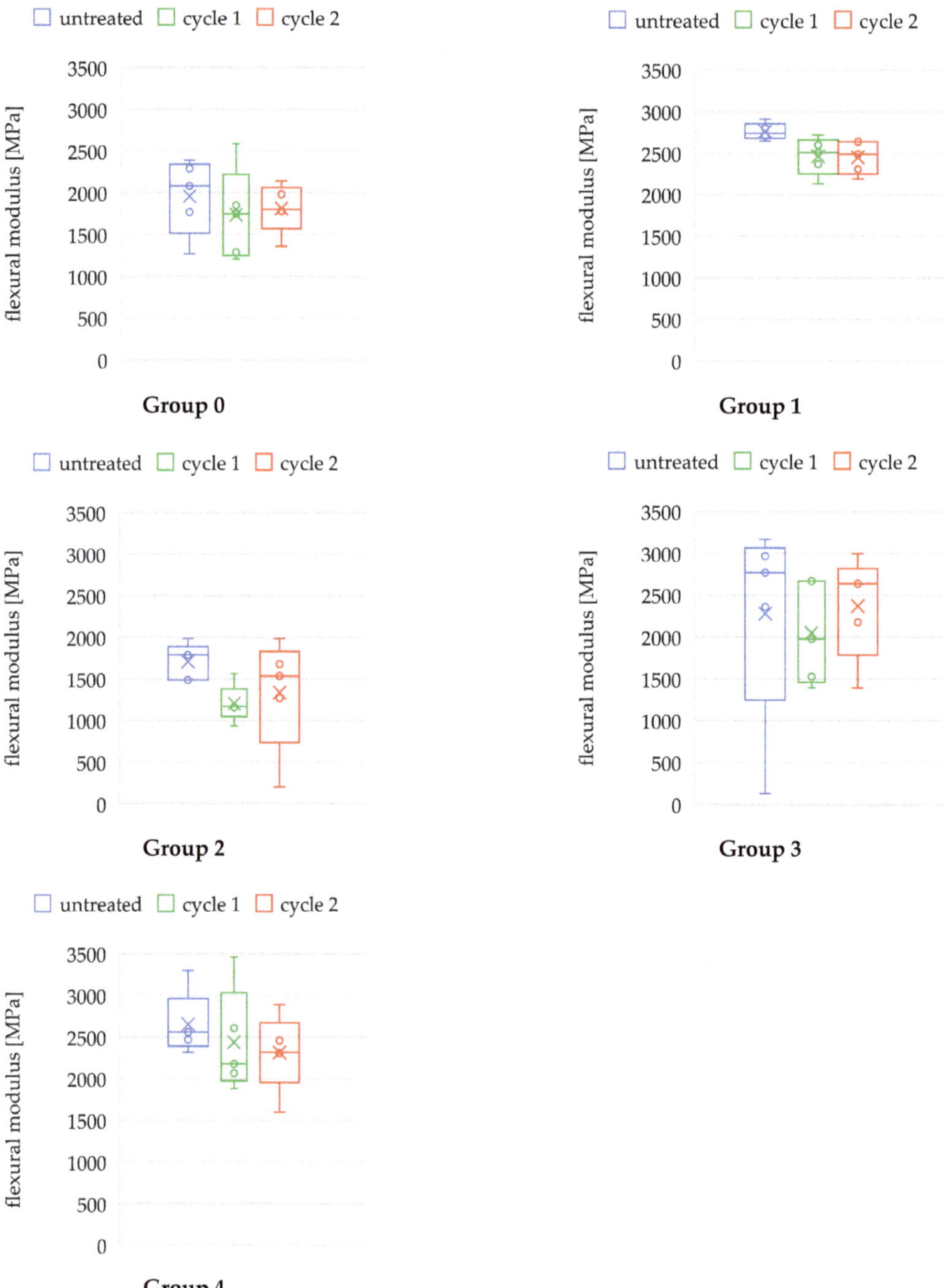

Figure 4. Boxplots: flexural moduli of the different groups and subgroups. The x represents the mean, the circles represent data points not covered by the boxplots.

4. Discussion

The aim of this study was to evaluate whether autoclaving changes the Vickers hardness and flexural modulus of resin materials used to additively manufacture insertion guides, which could pose a risk for the accuracy of static navigated implantation.

For the majority of specimens, the two autoclaving protocols had a minor impact on the flexural modulus, whereas changes in the Vickers hardness were more pronounced.

Looking at the results of the Vickers hardness testing, it seems that choosing the right autoclaving cycle might decrease the risk of hardness deterioration of the templates. In one out of the three groups exhibiting significant autoclaving-induced changes in the Vickers hardness (group 2), these changes occurred after the cycle 2 sterilization protocol (134 °C, 2 bar for 5.5 min) and not with the so-called "delicate" program cycle 1 (121 °C, 1 bar for 20.5 min). Overall, none of the materials that are authorized for autoclaving by the manufacturers showed signs of decreasing Vickers hardness after being autoclaved with cycle 1. Still, it is questionable whether the increase in hardness could be accompanied by a contraction of the material, which could lead to dimensional changes of the templates.

Our results showed that in most cases, autoclaving does not significantly change the flexural modulus of resin materials used to print the templates. Thus, it seems that autoclaving might not be a major risk factor for implantation accuracy loss caused by significant changes in the flexural modulus. We found no significant changes in the flexural modulus for groups 2, 3, and 4.

Interestingly, a decrease in flexural modulus was also seen in group 0, which was expected to be more prone to heat-induced changes in the flexural properties, as that resin is not authorized for autoclaving. Nevertheless, for most of the groups, the flexural moduli decreased to some extent. In group 1, autoclaving significantly decreased the flexural modulus, independently from the cycle.

Avoiding medical risks related to the contamination of the surgical site is the primary reason that makes autoclaving a must. It has been shown that the immersion in different disinfection solutions such as chlorhexidine digluconate, sodium hypochlorite, sodium perborate, or glutaraldehyde cannot entirely eradicate the microbial contamination of surgical template surfaces made of acrylic resin [31,32]. Ethanol at 70–80% resulted to be most effective among the disinfectants [25,32]. Tallarico et al. found that, after immersion disinfection with 70% ethanol for 15 min, about 16% of colony-forming units (CFU) remained on the resin surfaces [25]. Hence, in accordance with the risk mitigation when utilizing medical devices, as requested by the EU Medical Device Regulation [6], the sole reduction in microorganisms on surgical template surfaces by immersion disinfection seems insufficient and sterilization should be chosen. In light of our findings, the biological benefit of autoclaving the templates outweighs the risk of changes in the flexural properties or Vickers hardness. Nevertheless, some authors suggest cold sterilization protocols for heat-sensitive resin materials, i.e., utilizing ethylene oxide gas [33], which, however, are not commonly utilized in dental practice. The investigation of high-temperature sterilizing protocols such as autoclaving is clinically relevant, as it is one of the most commonly used methods in dentistry [34–37].

In agreement with our results for groups 1, 2, and 4, a pilot study by Török et al. found that additively manufactured template materials did not significantly change in hardness when subjected to 121 °C autoclaving [27]. Our observations differ to some extent, as we found significant changes of the hardness for group 3 after 121 °C autoclaving. Furthermore, their investigation on specimens that had been autoclaved at 134 °C exhibited significant changes in hardness values compared to specimens that were left untreated. These results are in line with our findings for groups 0 and 2. Despite utilizing similar autoclaving cycles (i.e., 121 °C, 1 bar, 20 min and 134 °C, 2 bar, 10 min), the varying observations could be a consequence of the different specimen preparation. In their work, the specimens were cut out of surgical templates, embedded, and coated with a gold layer to improve the visibility of the indentations prior to testing. In addition, the group conducted their tests with different parameters in terms of load (50 g) and duration (5 s). Furthermore, they investigated the flexural properties by testing for changes in the flexural strength, showing that autoclaving at 134 °C increased the materials stiffness significantly, while there were no significant changes in the flexural properties after autoclaving at 121 °C. Overall, our results are not entirely comparable, as different flexural properties were tested. Still, the results found in our study show similarities to the findings of Török et al., as we found no significant changes in the flexural modulus for 121 °C, while detecting a significant change for one group after autoclaving at 134 °C. However, the limited amount of data does not allow us to draw any firm conclusions about the influence of the autoclaving parameters on the flexural properties. It would be interesting to clarify whether autoclaving-induced changes in flexural properties are minor at lower sterilization temperature and pressure [27].

Most recently, Pop et al. conducted a similar study on the influence of disinfection and autoclaving on the flexural properties of surgical guide materials for additive manufacturing [29]. In contrast to our results, they found significantly increased flexural moduli for both autoclaving cycles that the specimens were subjected to (i.e., 121 °C, 1 bar, 20 min and 134 °C, 2 bar, 10 min). Reasons for the contrasting results could be different post-curing conditions of the specimens, different materials, different loading speed (i.e., 5 mm/s), and possibly different specimen geometry, which, however, remained unspecified. Interestingly, one of the two materials that were examined in their study was used in the present study in group 3 (i.e., Dental SG, Formlabs Inc.), which was the only group that we found to have an increased flexural modulus after being treated at 134 °C, in agreement with the results of Pop et al. [29].

Bayarsaikhan et al. investigated the behavior of resin materials for additive manufacturing when subjected to different temperatures (i.e., 40 °C, 60 °C, and 80 °C) and for varying treatment durations (i.e., 15, 30, 60, 90, and 120 min) after curing. They found that, with increasing temperature and treatment duration, the flexural modulus and Vickers hardness increased [30]. Jindal et al. conducted a resembling study on post-curing treatment, showing that 3D-printed aligner materials treated with higher temperatures endured higher compressive loads without deforming plastically [38].

In the present study, only two sterilization protocols were selected, and this might represent a limitation of the current study. However, the chosen protocols are among the simplest and most effective ones in dental practices and therefore are clinically relevant [39]. Another limitation is that not all the resin/printer combinations available on the market could be tested. Further, as recommended in the literature, specimens designed for mechanical testing were utilized, which is not 100% transferable to clinical settings. In addition, it has to be noted that three resins were printed with DLP, whereas only one resin was printed with SLA and SLA-LCD. It might be of interest to perform chemical analyses of the different materials before and after steam autoclaving to verify if there is any common pattern in autoclaving-induced chemical modifications. In future studies, in addition to the analysis of the mechanical properties, it would also be relevant to further explore the autoclaving-induced dimensional changes of templates fabricated by common resin–printer combinations.

5. Conclusions

In conclusion, and within the limitations of this study, in three groups out of five, a significant change in Vickers hardness was observed following autoclaving. This included the material not authorized for steam autoclaving. Just one material presented a significant decrease in the flexural modulus after cycle 2, whereas none of the materials showed a significant change following cycle 1. Thus, clinicians might consider using lower temperatures and pressures and longer autoclaving durations to sterilize additively manufactured templates. Materials authorized for autoclaving should be preferred. It is not possible to draw firm conclusions on the clinical significance of autoclaving-induced guide changes relying solely on biomechanical data. Indeed, whether and to what extent the autoclaving cycles are also associated with dimensional changes of the templates should be investigated in future studies.

Author Contributions: Conceptualization, K.B.; methodology, A.K., S.D., C.B. and K.B.; formal analysis, A.K. and K.B.; investigation, A.K. and L.K.; resources, S.D., C.B. and K.B.; data curation, K.B.; writing—original draft preparation, A.K., G.B. and K.B.; writing—review and editing, A.K., G.B., D.D. and K.B.; supervision, K.B.; project administration, K.B. All authors have read and agreed to the published version of the manuscript.

Funding: This research received no external funding.

Institutional Review Board Statement: Not applicable.

Informed Consent Statement: Not applicable.

Data Availability Statement: Data will be provided upon reasonable request.

Acknowledgments: The specimens printed with the materials NextDent SG, Vertex-Dental B.V., and Optiprint Guide, dentona AG were provided free of cost by Dentalstudio-Sankt Augustin GmbH. The other specimens were provided by 3D Agency oHG at a reduced cost. The authors would like to thank Viktoria Trelenberg-Stoll for her help in the conception of the study.

Conflicts of Interest: The authors declare no conflict of interest.

References

1. Louvrier, A.; Marty, P.; Barrabé, A.; Euvrard, E.; Chatelain, B.; Weber, E.; Meyer, C. How useful is 3D printing in maxillofacial surgery? *J. Stomatol. Oral Maxillofac. Surg.* **2017**, *118*, 206–212. [CrossRef] [PubMed]
2. Tattan, M.; Chambrone, L.; González-Martín, O.; Avila-Ortiz, G. Static computer-aided, partially guided, and free-handed implant placement: A systematic review and meta-analysis of randomized controlled trials. *Clin. Oral Implant. Res.* **2020**, *31*, 889–916. [CrossRef] [PubMed]
3. Chen, S.; Ou, Q.; Lin, X.; Wang, Y. Comparison between a Computer-Aided Surgical Template and the Free-Hand Method: A Systematic Review and Meta-Analysis. *Implant Dent.* **2019**, *28*, 578–589. [CrossRef] [PubMed]
4. Tahmaseb, A.; Wu, V.; Wismeijer, D.; Coucke, W.; Evans, C. The accuracy of static computer-aided implant surgery: A systematic review and meta-analysis. *Clin. Oral Implant. Res.* **2018**, *29*, 416–435. [CrossRef] [PubMed]
5. Lal, K.; White, G.S.; Morea, D.N.; Wright, R.F. Use of stereolithographic templates for surgical and prosthodontic implant planning and placement. Part I. The concept. *J. Prosthodont.* **2006**, *15*, 51–58. [CrossRef]
6. Regulation (EU) 2017/745 of the European Parliament and of the Council of 5 April 2017 on Medical Devices, Amending Directive 2001/83/EC, Regulation (EC) No 178/2002 and Regulation (EC) No 1223/2009 and Repealing Council Directives 90/385/EEC and 93/42/EEC. Annex 1, Chapters 1, 8. Available online: https://eur-lex.europa.eu/eli/reg/2017/745/oj (accessed on 16 February 2022).
7. Raico Gallardo, Y.N.; da Silva-Olivio, I.; Mukai, E.; Morimoto, S.; Sesma, N.; Cordaro, L. Accuracy comparison of guided surgery for dental implants according to the tissue of support: A systematic review and meta-analysis. *Clin. Oral Implant. Res.* **2017**, *28*, 602–612. [CrossRef] [PubMed]
8. Cassetta, M.; Stefanelli, L.V.; Giansanti, M.; Di Mambro, A.; Calasso, S. Depth deviation and occurrence of early surgical complications or unexpected events using a single stereolithographic surgi-guide. *J. Stomatol. Oral Maxillofac. Surg.* **2011**, *40*, 1377–1387. [CrossRef]
9. Schnutenhaus, S.; Edelmann, C.; Rudolph, H.; Luthardt, R.G. Retrospective study to determine the accuracy of template-guided implant placement using a novel nonradiologic evaluation method. *Oral Surg. Oral Med. Oral Pathol. Oral Radiol.* **2016**, *121*, 72–79. [CrossRef]
10. Makins, S.R. Artifacts interfering with interpretation of cone beam computed tomography images. *Dent. Clin. N. Am.* **2014**, *58*, 485–495. [CrossRef]
11. Tadinada, A.; Jalali, E.; Jadhav, A.; Schincaglia, G.P.; Yadav, S. Artifacts in Cone Beam Computed Tomography Image Volumes: An Illustrative Depiction. *J. Mass. Dent. Soc.* **2015**, *64*, 12–15.
12. Giménez, B.; Özcan, M.; Martínez-Rus, F.; Pradíes, G. Accuracy of a digital impression system based on active wavefront sampling technology for implants considering operator experience, implant angulation, and depth. *Clin. Implant Dent. Relat. Res.* **2015**, *17*, 54–64. [CrossRef] [PubMed]
13. Joda, T.; Zarone, F.; Ferrari, M. The complete digital workflow in fixed prosthodontics: A systematic review. *BMC Oral Health* **2017**, *17*, 124. [CrossRef] [PubMed]
14. Cassetta, M.; Giansanti, M.; Di Mambro, A.; Stefanelli, L.V. Accuracy of positioning of implants inserted using a mucosa-supported stereolithographic surgical guide in the edentulous maxilla and mandible. *Int. J. Oral Maxillofac. Implant.* **2014**, *29*, 1071–1078. [CrossRef] [PubMed]

15. El Kholy, K.; Janner, S.F.M.; Schimmel, M.; Buser, D. The influence of guided sleeve height, drilling distance, and drilling key length on the accuracy of static computer-assisted implant surgery. *Clin. Implant Dent. Relat. Res.* **2019**, *21*, 101–107. [CrossRef] [PubMed]

16. Cassetta, M.; Altieri, F.; Di Giorgio, R.; Barbato, E. Palatal orthodontic miniscrew insertion using a CAD-CAM surgical guide: Description of a technique. *Int. J. Clin. Oral Maxillofac. Surg.* **2018**, *47*, 1195–1198. [CrossRef] [PubMed]

17. Jedliński, M.; Janiszewska-Olszowska, J.; Mazur, M.; Ottolenghi, L.; Grocholewicz, K.; Galluccio, G. Guided Insertion of Temporary Anchorage Device in Form of Orthodontic Titanium Miniscrews with Customized 3D Templates—A Systematic Review with Meta-Analysis of Clinical Studies. *Coatings* **2021**, *11*, 1488. [CrossRef]

18. Becker, K.; Unland, J.; Wilmes, B.; Tarraf, N.E.; Drescher, D. Is there an ideal insertion angle and position for orthodontic mini-implants in the anterior palate? A CBCT study in humans. *Am. J. Orthod. Dentofac. Orthop.* **2019**, *156*, 345–354. [CrossRef]

19. Küffer, M.; Drescher, D.; Becker, K. Application of the Digital Workflow in Orofacial Orthopedics and Orthodontics: Printed Appliances with Skeletal Anchorage. *J. Appl. Sci.* **2022**, *12*, 3820. [CrossRef]

20. D'haese, J.; Ackhurst, J.; Wismeijer, D.; De Bruyn, H.; Tahmaseb, A. Current state of the art of computer-guided implant surgery. *Periodontology 2000* **2017**, *73*, 121–133. [CrossRef]

21. Wegmüller, L.; Halbeisen, F.; Sharma, N.; Kühl, S.; Thieringer, F.M. Consumer vs. High-End 3D Printers for Guided Implant Surgery-An In Vitro Accuracy Assessment Study of Different 3D Printing Technologies. *J. Clin. Med.* **2021**, *10*, 4894. [CrossRef]

22. Herschdorfer, L.; Negreiros, W.M.; Gallucci, G.O.; Hamilton, A. Comparison of the accuracy of implants placed with CAD-CAM surgical templates manufactured with various 3D printers: An in vitro study. *J. Prosthet. Dent.* **2021**, *125*, 905–910. [CrossRef] [PubMed]

23. Chen LLin, W.S.; Polido, W.D.; Eckert, G.J.; Morton, D. Accuracy, reproducibility, and dimensional stability of additively manufactured surgical templates. *J. Prosthet. Dent.* **2019**, *122*, 309–314. [CrossRef] [PubMed]

24. Kohn, W.G.; Collins, A.S.; Cleveland, J.L.; Harte, J.A.; Eklund, K.J.; Malvitz, D.M.; Centers for Disease Control and Prevention (CDC). Guidelines for infection control in dental health-care settings—2003. *MMWR Recomm. Rep.* **2003**, *52*, 1–61. [PubMed]

25. Tallarico, M.; Lumbau, A.I.; Park, C.J.; Puddu, A.; Sanseverino, F.; Amarena, R.; Meloni, S.M. In vitro evaluation of biodburden, three-dimensional stability, and accuracy of surgical templates without metallic sleeves after routinely infection control activities. *Clin. Implant Dent. Relat. Res.* **2021**, *23*, 380–387. [CrossRef] [PubMed]

26. Marei, H.F.; Alshaia, A.; Alarifi, S.; Almasoud, N.; Abdelhady, A. Effect of Steam Heat Sterilization on the Accuracy of 3D Printed Surgical Guides. *Implant Dent.* **2019**, *28*, 372–377. [CrossRef]

27. Török, G.; Gombocz, P.; Bognár, E.; Nagy, P.; Dinya, E.; Kispélyi, B.; Hermann, P. Effects of disinfection and sterilization on the dimensional changes and mechanical properties of 3D printed surgical guides for implant therapy—Pilot study. *BMC Oral Health* **2020**, *20*, 19. [CrossRef]

28. Quintana, R.; Choi, J.W.; Puebla, K.; Wicker, R. Effects of build orientation on tensile strength for stereolithography-manufactured ASTM D-638 type I specimens. *Int. J. Adv. Manuf. Technol.* **2010**, *46*, 201–215. [CrossRef]

29. Pop, S.I.; Dudescu, M.; Mihali, S.G.; Păcurar, M.; Bratu, D.C. Effects of Disinfection and Steam Sterilization on the Mechanical Properties of 3D SLA- and DLP-Printed Surgical Guides for Orthodontic Implant Placement. *Polymers* **2022**, *14*, 2107. [CrossRef]

30. Bayarsaikhan, E.; Lim, J.H.; Shin, S.H.; Park, K.H.; Park, Y.B.; Lee, J.H.; Kim, J.E. Effects of Postcuring Temperature on the Mechanical Properties and Biocompatibility of Three-Dimensional Printed Dental Resin Material. *Polymers* **2021**, *13*, 1180. [CrossRef]

31. Da Silva, F.C.; Kimpara, E.T.; Mancini, M.N.; Balducci, I.; Jorge, A.O.; Koga-Ito, C.Y. Effectiveness of six different disinfectants on removing five microbial species and effects on the topographic characteristics of acrylic resin. *J. Prosthodont.* **2008**, *17*, 627–633. [CrossRef]

32. Sennhenn-Kirchner, S.; Weustermann, S.; Mergeryan, H.; Jacobs, H.G.; Borg-von Zepelin, M.; Kirchner, B. Preoperative sterilization and disinfection of drill guide templates. *Clin. Oral Investig.* **2008**, *12*, 179–187. [CrossRef] [PubMed]

33. Smith, P.N.; Palenik, C.J.; Blanchard, S.B. Microbial contamination and the sterilization/disinfection of surgical guides used in the placement of endosteal implants. *Int. J. Oral Maxillofac. Implant.* **2011**, *26*, 274–281.

34. Smith, A.J.; Bagg, J.; Hurrell, D.; McHugh, S. Sterilization of re-usable instruments in general dental practice. *Br. Dent. J.* **2007**, *203*, E16. [CrossRef] [PubMed]

35. Mahasneh, A.M.; Alakhras, M.; Khabour, O.F.; Al-Sa'di, A.G.; Al-Mousa, D.S. Practices of Infection Control among Dental Care Providers: A Cross Sectional Study. *Clin. Cosmet. Investig. Dent.* **2020**, *12*, 281–289. [CrossRef]

36. Dagher, J.; Sfeir, C.; Abdallah, A.; Majzoub, Z. Sterilization and Biologic Monitoring in Private Dental Clinics in Lebanon. *J. Contemp. Dent. Pract.* **2018**, *19*, 853–861.

37. Röhm-Rodowald, E.; Jakimiak, B.; Chojecka, A.; Zmuda-Baranowska, M.; Kanclerski, K. Ocena procesów dekontaminacji: Mycia, dezynfekcji i sterylizacji w praktyce stomatologicznej w Polsce w latach 2011–2012 [Assessment of decontamination processes: Cleaning, disinfection and sterilization in dental practice in Poland in the years 2011–2012]. *Prz. Epidemiol.* **2012**, *66*, 635–641.

38. Jindal, P.; Juneja, M.; Bajaj, D.; Siena, F.L.; Breedon, P. Effects of post-curing conditions on mechanical properties of 3D printed clear dental aligners. *Rapid Prototyp. J.* **2020**, *26*, 1337–1344. [CrossRef]

39. Jakubovics, N.; Greenwood, M.; Meechan, J.G. General medicine and surgery for dental practitioners: Part 4. Infections and infection control. *Br. Dent. J.* **2014**, *217*, 73–77. [CrossRef]

 *applied sciences*

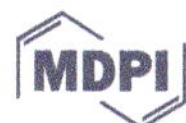

Article

Impact of Dental Model Height on Thermoformed PET-G Aligner Thickness—An In Vitro Micro-CT Study

Benjamin Alexander Ihssen [1,2,†], Robert Kerberger [1,†], Nicole Rauch [3], Dieter Drescher [1] and Kathrin Becker [1,*]

1   Department of Orthodontics, University of Düsseldorf, 40225 Düsseldorf, Germany; benjamin.ihssen@googlemail.com (B.A.I.); Robert.kerberger@med.uni-duesseldorf.de (R.K.); drescher@med.uni-duesseldorf.de (D.D.)

2   Private Practice, 31224 Peine, Germany

3   Department of Oral Surgery, University of Düsseldorf, 40225 Düsseldorf, Germany; Nicole.rauch@med.uni-duesseldorf.de

*   Correspondence: kathrin.becker@med.uni-duesseldorf.de; Tel.: +49-211-811-81-45

†   Both authors contributed equally.

Abstract: The aim of the present study was to investigate whether base height of 3D-printed dental models has an impact on local thickness values from polyethylene terephthalate glycol (PET-G) aligners. A total of 20 aligners were thermoformed on dental models from the upper jaw exhibiting either a 5 mm high (H) or narrow (N), i.e., 0 mm, base height. The aligners were digitized using micro-CT, segmented, and local thickness values were computed utilizing a 3D-distance transform. The mean thickness values and standard deviations were assessed for both groups, and local thickness values at pre-defined reference points were also recorded. The statistical analysis was performed using R. Aligners in group H were significantly thinner and more homogenous compared to group N ($p < 0.001$). Significant differences in thickness values were observed among tooth types between both groups. Whereas thickness values were comparable at cusp tips and occlusal/incisal/cervical measurement locations, facial and palatal surfaces were significantly thicker in group N compared to group H ($p < 0.01$). Within the limits of the study, the base height of 3D-printed models impacts on local thickness values of thermoformed aligners. The clinician should consider potential implication on exerted forces at the different tooth types, and at facial as well as palatal surfaces.

Keywords: aligner; Micro-CT; PETG; thermoforming; material characteristics

Citation: Ihssen, B.A.; Kerberger, R.; Rauch, N.; Drescher, D.; Becker, K. Impact of Dental Model Height on Thermoformed PET-G Aligner Thickness—An In Vitro Micro-CT Study. *Appl. Sci.* **2021**, *11*, 6674. https://doi.org/10.3390/app11156674

Academic Editor: Giuliana Muzio

Received: 18 June 2021
Accepted: 15 July 2021
Published: 21 July 2021

Publisher's Note: MDPI stays neutral with regard to jurisdictional claims in published maps and institutional affiliations.

1. Introduction

Aligners, thermoformed from elastic polymers, gained widespread application in recent years [1,2] due to ease of use, patient comfort, aesthetics, ease of oral hygiene and a reduced risk for white spot lesions [3–5].

Despite their broad application, predictability of aligner treatment outcomes is still controversially discussed [6–8]. Discrepancies between the initial setup and final outcomes may owe to patient related factors (patient adherence, metabolic factors), and may also relate to inaccurate prediction of the force systems exerted on teeth [9]. Even though initially neglected, side effects from orthodontic treatment occur not only with fixed appliances, but also in aligner therapy [10,11]. Especially forces of higher magnitude and uncontrolled tipping of teeth have to be avoided in order to limit root resorption [12,13]. Thus, improving biomechanical understanding of exerted forces and moments is of crucial importance to enhance safety and predictability of aligner treatments.

In-vitro studies demonstrated that initial forces and moments of aligners can exceed recommended force levels up to the factor six [14–17]. As reported earlier, force magnitudes can be decreased by utilizing thinner aligner raw materials [18,19]. However, the final thicknesses of aligners depend on the thermoforming process and might be associated with geometric properties of the 3D-printed dental cast employed for manufacturing. Furthermore, as 3D-printed aligners are still rarely used, and as thermoforming is frequently manually conducted by a trained technician, aligners may not be perfectly homogenous even if they are fabricated on the same cast [20].

Few techniques exist to assess homogeneity and microstructure of thermoplastic materials. Micro-computed tomography (micro-CT), whose laboratory usage has been introduced in the 1990s for structural analysis of calcified tissues, provides high resolution three-dimensional images from various specimen [21]. Its applicability to assess aligner material properties has been demonstrated recently [22–25].

Therefore, the present study aimed at assessing the impact of dental model height on PET-G aligner thickness values, and at investigating the within-group variability of thickness values potentially arising from the manual fabrication process.

2. Materials and Methods

2.1. Study Design

The present study reports on a sample of n = 20 polyethylene terephthalate glycol (PET-G) aligners. The aligners were thermoformed on a 3D-printed dental model of the upper jaw with either narrow (N) base height, or high (H) base height (achieved by placing a spacer of 5 mm height) (n = 10 aligners per group, respectively). The perpendicular distance between occlusal plane and model-tray were defined as model height and amounted to 11 mm (Figure 1). Consequently, model height in the N group was 11 mm, and 16 mm in the H group.

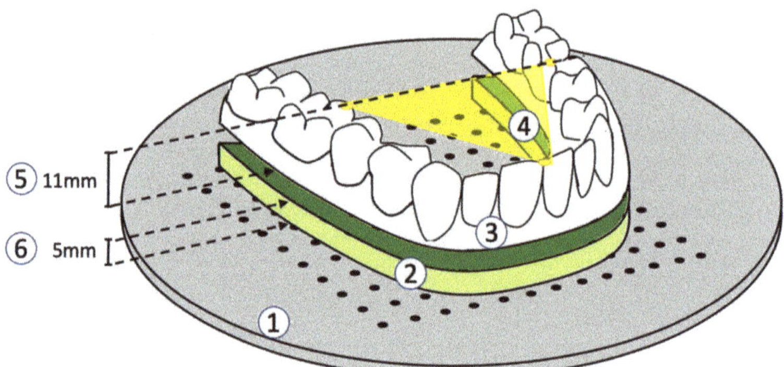

Figure 1. Thermoforming-Setup (1: model tray; 2: spacer; 3: acrylic dental arch model; 4: occlusal plane parallel to the model tray; 5: model height = 11 mm; 6: spacer height = 5 mm).

The 3d-printed model was fabricated using a SLA printer (Form 2, Formlabs Inc., Somerville, MA, USA) at 100 micron resolution (100% infill) and using the Draft Resin (Formlabs Inc.). The model was oriented in a nearly vertical position to minimize warping. The model was manually cleaned and cured according to manufacturer's recommendations. After curing, the model base was manually grinded to compensate any warping and ensure full flat contact to the thermoforming tray. It was then stored at ambient air at 20 °C and 50% humidity.

2.2. Thermoforming

Thermoforming was achieved using a Biostar thermoforming machine (Biostar VII, Scheu Dental, Iserlohn, Germany) and a PET-G raw material of 0.5 mm thickness (CA Clear Aligner, Scheu Dental, Iserlohn, Germany). The dental model was placed in the center of the thermoforming chamber such that the mid palatal suture was located in 12 o'clock position. The occlusal plane was oriented parallel to a perforated custom model-tray (Figure 1). The dental model was held in place by 3 positioning pins to ensure constant localization and orientation for each thermoforming process.

Settings for heating and pressure forming were the same for all aligners (21 °C ambient air, 50% humidity, 20 s, 220 °C). The edges of all aligners were trimmed to a line 1 mm cervically of the gingival margin after thermoforming.

2.3. Micro-Computed Tomography and Image Processing

All aligners were scanned with a micro-CT scanner (VivaCT 80, Scanco Medical AG, Wangen-Brüttisellen, Switzerland). The scans were performed at 45 kVp, 88 µA, and 254 ms integration time and reconstructed to a nominal isotropic voxel size of 31.2 µm.

Image processing was performed using an in-house programmed script implemented with the Image Processing Language (IPL) (Scanco Medical AG, Wangen-Brüttisellen, Switzerland) which performed the following steps:

First, a cylindric volume of interest (VOI) was placed at the outer margin of the field of view. Then, a threshold of 4.2% was used to segment the aligners within VOI. Aligner thickness was then calculated by means of the 3D-Chamfer-Distance transform approach [26]. In brief, this approach calculates the outer contours of a segmented material and it assigns the Euclidean distance to its closest contour point as grey value to every point within the segmented structure. Hence, zero values represent contour points, whereas higher values represent greater thickness values. For visualization purposes, the calculated aligner thickness values were eventually rendered using a 3D-rendering program (uct_3d, Scanco Medical AG, Wangen-Brüttisellen, Switzerland) (Figure 2).

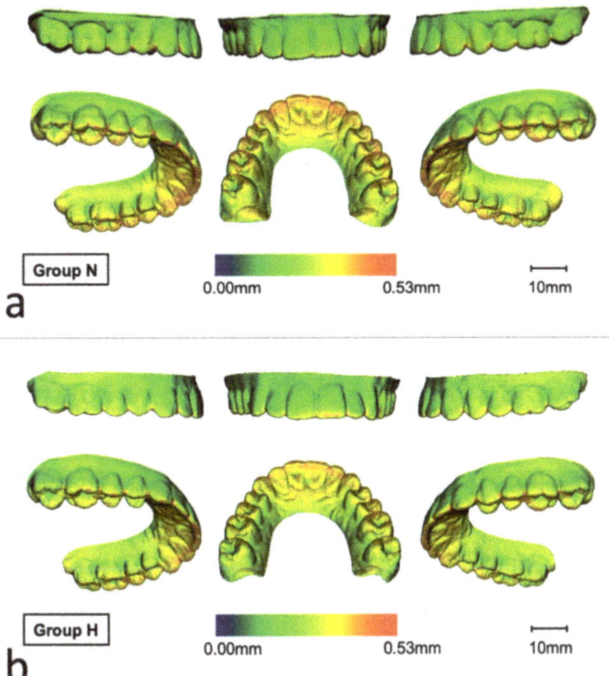

Figure 2. Representative renderings visualizing the local material thickness of micro-CT scanned aligners thermoformed at (**a**) narrow (N) or (**b**) heigh (H) dental models (blue: 0.00 mm, red: 0.53 mm). Thickness values were higher in the N group compared to the H group, especially in the anterior palatal area, occlusally and on incisal edges.

2.4. Thickness Measurements

To assess local aligner thickness values, a total of n = 29 reference points were utilized (Table 1). At each reference point, the respective local thickness was recorded.

Table 1. Reference points for assessment of local aligner material thickness values. The column "aggregated location" specifies which values were aggregated per group (high/narrow) or tooth type (molar/premolar/canine/front), respectively. The right column specifies the teeth at which the thickness measurements were recorded.

Reference Point	Definition	Aggregated Location	Assessed at Teeth
MB	mesiobuccal cusp tip		16, 26
DB	distobuccal cusp tip		16, 26
B	buccal cusp tip	Cusp tip	15, 14, 25, 24
MP	mesiopalatal cusp tip		16, 26
DP	distopalatal cusp tip		16, 26
P	palatal cusp tip		15, 14, 25, 24
FIS	mesiodistal center of the central fissure	Occlusal	16, 15, 14, 26, 25, 24
I	most coronal, central point of the incisal edge	Incisal	11, 21, 12, 22, 13, 23
FLA	LA-Point of the facial surface	Facial	All teeth
FC	most cervical point of the vestibular surface	Facial-cervical	All teeth
PLA	LA-Point of the palatal surface	Palatal	All teeth
PC	most cervical point of the palatal surface	Palatal-cervical	All teeth

2.5. Statistical Analysis

The statistical analysis was performed using R 2021 [26]. To compare the mean thickness values and the respective standard deviations between N and H groups, the Mann-Whitney-U test was used.

For descriptive purposes, local thickness values at reference points were aggregated for the variables tooth type (molar/premolar/canine/front) and measurement location (Table 1) and presented as boxplots.

To assess the relationship between thickness values and the effects tooth type/measurement location, the lme4-package [27] was used to perform linear mixed effects models. As fixed effects, we entered tooth type and measurement location (with and without interaction term) into the model. As random effects, we had intercepts for aligners. Visual inspection of residual plots did not reveal any obvious deviations from homoscedasticity or normality. p-values were obtained by likelihood ratio tests of the full model with the effect in question against the model without the effect in question. Post-hoc tests were conducted using the emmeans-package [28], and the Tukey-method was utilized for p-value correction. The results were found significant at $p < 0.05$.

3. Results

The in-house developed script enabled successful automated segmentation of the aligners. Calculation of the distance transform enabled assessment of thickness values (Figure 2).

3.1. Comparison of Thickness Values

Mean thickness values were significantly lower in group H compared to N (median [quartile 1–3]: 0.30 [0.30–0.30] vs. 0.32 [0.31–0.32], $p < 0.001$). When comparing the standard deviations, which correspond to material homogeneity, values in group H were significantly lower compared to group N (median [1st–3rd quartile]: 0.064 [0.063–0.65] vs. 0.061 [0.060–0.062], $p < 0.001$) (Figure 3).

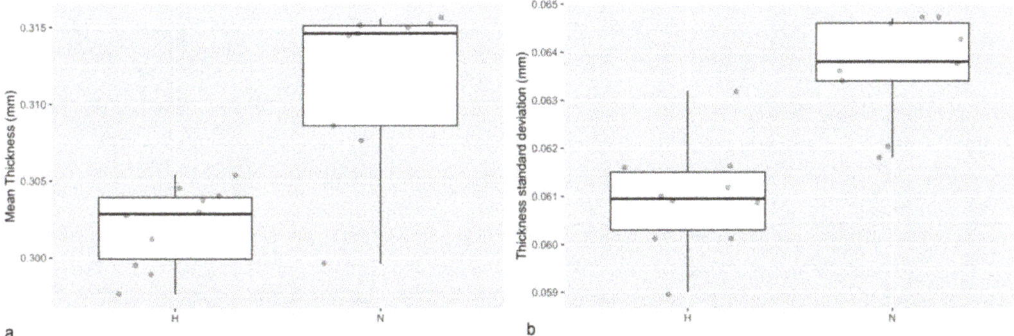

Figure 3. (**a**) Boxplot showing the mean thickness values of aligners thermoformed at narrow (N) and high (H) dental models. (**b**) Boxplot showing the standard deviation of the respective thickness values representing the material homogeneity.

3.2. Comparison of Local Thickness Values at Selected Tooth Types

To assess whether the tooth type has an impact on the material thickness, a linear mixed effects model was used. A significant effect of the effects group and tooth type were found ($p < 0.001$, respectively), and also the interaction of group (high vs. narrow) and tooth type was found to be significant ($p < 0.001$). Thickness values were higher in N group, and differences between tooth types were also more pronounced in N group (Figure 4).

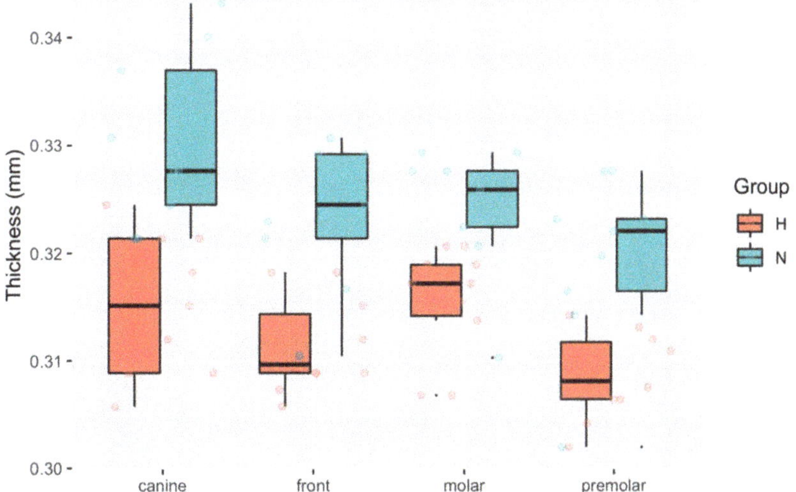

Figure 4. Boxplot showing the local thickness values at reference points for group high (H) and narrow (N). The thickness values at the reference points were aggregated by tooth type. Thickness values were higher in the N compared to the H group ($p < 0.001$), and highest values were seen at canines in the N group.

The post hoc test revealed significant differences between groups for each tooth type, and the estimated difference was greatest at canines (Table 2). Within-group multiple comparison revealed significant differences between premolars and canines or premolars in the H-group, and canine versus front teeth or premolars in the N-group (Table 3).

Table 2. Estimated mean [standard error (SE)] for the local thickness values (mm) from group high (H) and narrow (N) aggregated by tooth type. Comparison was achieved using multiple comparison post hoc test with Tukey-method for p-value adjustment (family of 8 estimates). ** $p < 0.01$, *** $p < 0.001$.

	Estimate (SE) Group H	Estimate (SE) Group N	Est. Difference (SE)	p-Value
Molar	0.316 (0.002)	0.324 (0.002)	−0.003 (0.003)	0.077 **
Premolar	0.309 (0.002)	0.320 (0.002)	−0.011 (0.003)	0.007 **
Canine	0.315 (0.002)	0.330 (0.002)	−0.015 (0.003)	<0.001 ***
Front	0.311 (0.002)	0.323 (0.002)	−0.012 (0.003)	0.002 **

Table 3. Within-group comparison of local thickness values (mm) for group high (H) and narrow (N) aggregated for tooth type. Comparison was achieved using multiple comparison post hoc test with Tukey-method for p-value adjustment (family of 4 estimates), respectively. * $p < 0.05$, ** $p < 0.01$, *** $p < 0.001$.

	Comparison	Estimated Difference (SE)	T-Ratio	p-Value
Group H	canine–front	0.003 (0.003)	1.903	0.251
	canine–molar	−0.001 (0.003)	−0.571	0.940
	canine–premolar	0.006 (0.003)	3.545	0.008 **
	front–molar	−0.004 (0.002)	−2.561	0.074
	front–premolar	0.003 (0.002)	1.700	0.344
	molar–premolar	0.007 (0.002)	4.261	0.001 **
Group N	canine–front	0.007 (0.003)	2.770	0.044 *
	canine–molar	0.006 (0.003)	2.493	0.081
	canine–premolar	0.011 (0.003)	4.323	<0.001 ***
	front–molar	−0.001 (0.003)	−0.277	0.992
	front–premolar	0.004 (0.003)	1.553	0.420
	molar–premolar	0.006 (0.003)	1.830	0.279

3.3. Comparison of Thickness Values at Measurement Locations

Linear mixed effects models revealed a significant effect of group and measurement location ($p < 0.001$, respectively), as well as for their interaction ($p < 0.001$). Thickness values were slightly higher in N group at most of the locations. With respect to the measurement location, thickness values were smallest at facial surfaces and highest at incisal faces. Thickness values were also higher at cusp tips compared to the fissures (occlusal surface), and within a medium range at palatal surfaces (Figure 5).

Post-hoc multiple comparison revealed significant differences at facial and palatal surfaces (Table 4). Within-group comparison revealed significant differences between all measurement locations except palatal and palatal-cervical, respectively (Table 5).

Table 4. Between-group comparison of local thickness values (mm) from group high (H) and narrow (N) aggregated for measurement location. Comparison was achieved using a multiple comparison post hoc test with Tukey-method for p-value adjustment (family of 14 estimates), respectively. ** $p < 0.01$, *** $p < 0.001$.

Comparison	Est. (SE) Group H	Est. (SE) Group N	Est. Difference (SE)	p-Value
Cusp tip	0.372 (0.003)	0.384 (0.003)	−0.012 (0.004)	0.090
Occlusal	0.285 (0.003)	0.278 (0.003)	0.007 (0.004)	0.902
Incisal	0.427 (0.003)	0.434 (0.003)	−0.008 (0.004)	0.751
Facial	0.243 (0.003)	0.268 (0.003)	−0.025 (0.004)	<0.001 ***
Facial-cervical	0.222 (0.003)	0.224 (0.003)	−0.002 (0.004)	1.000
Palatal	0.332 (0.003)	0.347 (0.003)	−0.015 (0.004)	0.005 **
Palatal-cervical	0.327 (0.003)	0.339 (0.003)	−0.012 (0.004)	0.073

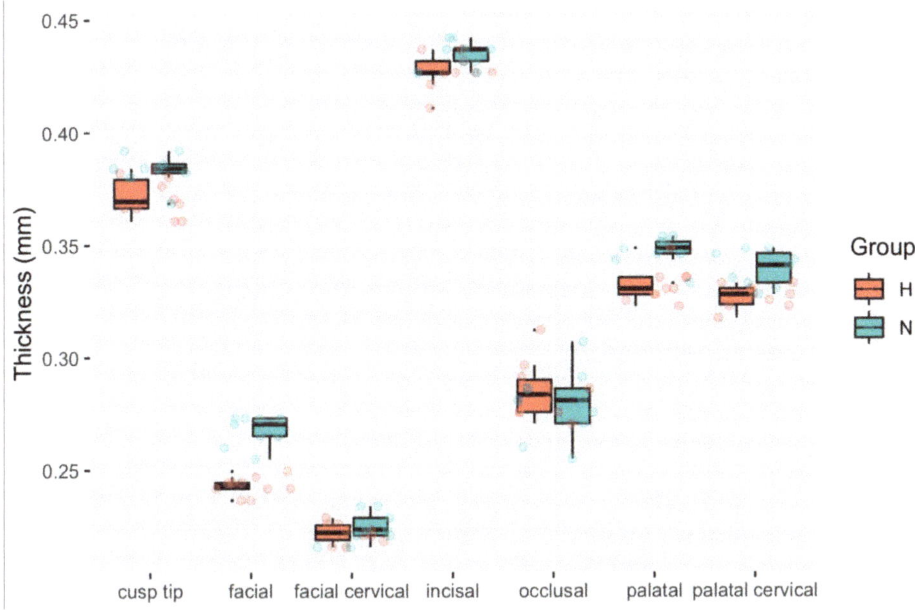

Figure 5. Boxplot showing the local thickness values at reference points for group high (H) and narrow (N). The local thickness values were aggregated by tooth measurement location. Highest values were seen at cusp tips, and palatal as well as palatal cervical faces.

Table 5. Within-group comparison of local thickness values (mm) for group high (H) and narrow (N) aggregated for measurement location. Comparison was achieved using multiple comparison post hoc test with Tukey-method for *p*-value adjustment (family of 7 estimates), respectively. * $p < 0.05$, *** $p < 0.001$.

	Comparison	Est. Difference (SE)	T-Ratio	*p*-Value
	cusp tip–facial	0.129 (0.003)	38.735	<0.001 ***
	cusp tip–facial cervical	0.150 (0.003)	44.989	<0.001 ***
	cusp tip–incisal	−0.055 (0.003)	−16.118	<0.001 ***
	cusp tip–occlusal	0.087 (0.003)	26.071	<0.001 ***
	cusp tip–palatal	0.040 (0.003)	12.000	<0.001 ***
	cusp tip–palatal cervical	0.045 (0.003)	13.485	<0.001 ***
	facial–facial cervical	0.021 (0.003)	6.254	<0.001 ***
	facial–incisal	−0.184 (0.003)	−53.726	<0. 001 ***
	facial–occlusal	−0.042 (0.003)	−12.664	<0.001 ***
Group H	facial–palatal	−0.089 (0.003)	−26.735	<0.001 ***
	facial–palatal cervical	−0.084 (0.003)	−25.250	<0.001 ***
	facial cervical–incisal	−0.205 (0.003)	−59.798	<0.001 ***
	facial cervical–occlusal	−0.063 (0.003)	−18.918	<0.001 ***
	facial cervical–palatal	−0.110 (0.003)	−32.989	<0.001 ***
	facial cervical–palatal cervical	−0.105 (0.003)	−31.504	<0.001 ***
	incisal–occlusal	0.142 (0.003)	41.431	<0.001 ***
	incisal–palatal	0.095 (0.003)	27.768	<0.001 ***
	incisal–palatal cervical	0.100 (0.003)	29.211	<0.001 ***
	occlusal–palatal	−0.047 (0.003)	−14.071	<0.001 ***
	occlusal–palatal cervical	−0.042 (0.003)	−12.586	<0.001 ***
	palatal–palatal cervical	0.005 (0.003)	1.485	0.752

Table 5. *Cont.*

	Comparison	Est. Difference (SE)	T-Ratio	*p*-Value
Group N	cusp tip–facial	0.116 (0.003)	35.565	<0.001 ***
	cusp tip–facial cervical	0.160 (0.003)	48.827	<0.001 ***
	cusp tip–incisal	−0.051 (0.003)	−15.539	<0.001 ***
	cusp tip–occlusal	0.105 (0.003)	32.205	<0.001 ***
	cusp tip–palatal	0.037 (0.003)	11.162	<0.001 ***
	cusp tip–palatal cervical	0.045 (0.003)	13.638	<0.001 ***
	facial–facial cervical	0.043 (0.003)	13.262	<0.001 ***
	facial–incisal	−0.167 (0.003)	−51.103	<0.001 ***
	facial–occlusal	−0.011 (0.003)	−3.360	0.022 *
	facial–palatal	−0.080 (0.003)	−24.402	<0.001 ***
	facial–palatal cervical	−0.072 (0.003)	−21.927	<0.001 ***
	facial cervical–incisal	−0.210 (0.003)	−64.366	<0.001 ***
	facial cervical–occlusal	−0.054 (0.003)	−16.622	<0.001 ***
	facial cervical–palatal	−0.123 (0.003)	−37.664	<0.001 ***
	facial cervical–palatal cervical	−0.115 (0.003)	−35.189	<0.001 ***
	incisal–occlusal	0.156 (0.003)	47.744	<0.001 ***
	incisal–palatal	0.087 (0.003)	26.701	<0.001 ***
	incisal–palatal cervical	0.100 (0.003)	29.177	<0.001 ***
	occlusal–palatal	−0.06875	−21.043	<0.001 ***
	occlusal–palatal cervical	−0.06067	−18.567	<0.001 ***
	palatal–palatal cervical	0.00809	2.476	0.187

4. Discussion

Previous research revealed that predictability and accuracy of aligner treatments can be as low as 30–50% when compared with the initial setup [14–17,29]. Besides patient related factors, varying material thickness of aligners has been suspected to impact on predictability of aligner treatments [18]. Therefore, the present study aimed at evaluating homogeneity of thermoformed PET-G aligners, and whether base height of 3D-printed dental models also impacts on material thickness values at different measurement locations.

The present study identified that aligners formed on narrow (N) models exhibited higher thickness values compared to those produced on higher (H) dental models. Material homogeneity was greater in the H compared to the N group. Additionally, thickness values varied with respect to the tooth types, and the measurement locations. Highest values were found at incisal edges and cusp tips, followed by palatal surfaces, and lowest values were seen at the facial aspects. Comparison between N and H groups did not reach statistical significance at most measurement locations. At palatal and facial surfaces, however, aligners from group N were significantly thicker compared to group H.

According to literature, the area moment of inertia is calculated using the third power of material diameter in direction of the acting forces [30]. Therefore, a 10% reduction of aligner material thickness could in theory reduce exerted forces up to 30%. In the present study, facial surfaces showed the smallest thickness values (estimated mean thickness group H/N: 0.243 mm/0.268 mm), whereas palatal (0.332 mm/0.347 mm) and incisal surfaces (0.427 mm/0.434 mm) showed highest values. Therefore, thickness values were 38–43% higher at incisal and 20–25% higher at palatal compared to facial surfaces. Differences between the groups amounted to 9% at the facial and 4% at palatal faces. Thus, these differences appear to be in a clinically relevant range, potentially impacting on treatment predictability.

Nonetheless, it must be noted that force transmission patterns from aligners are complex and not yet fully understood [31,32]. This owes to the so called "half shell shapes" of aligners and differences in localization of contact areas to teeth and attachments. Additionally, material deformation when aligners are put on the teeth, and material swelling due to saliva exposure must be considered. Therefore, aligner thickness is not the only factor influencing resulting forces and moments.

Scientific disagreement persists concerning the capability of aligners to perform bodily tooth movement [29,31,33,34], which necessitates application of a counterbalancing moment for control of root position [35]. In the present study, aligner specimens were thinnest at the facial/facial-cervical aspects, which is in line with a recent study revealing a 50% reduction of layer thickness in buccal-gingival regions [36]. Previous research demonstrated that low thickness values can lead to aligner deformation at the gingival margin [15], eventually resulting in reduced root control. However, besides the rigidity of aligners, application of attachments and shape modification like power buttons or ridges are also relevant to control tooth movement [32,37]. Thus, the impact of the facial/facial-gingival thinning should be further explored in future investigations.

The impact of dental model height has not been addressed in previous studies, despite its potential association with aligner thickness values, and therefore, the resulting force systems. In the present investigation, aligners thermoformed on the higher model showed increased homogeneity of material thickness values, but also a decreased overall thickness. Therefore, it may be speculated that adopting raw material thickness and height of 3D-printed models may be advantageous to better control the material thickness properties of thermoformed aligners, and eventually the resulting force systems. Additionally, as crown height varies among patients [38], clinicians should also carefully consider that higher crowns may lead to reduced thickness values, and vice versa.

Posterior bite opening is one of the common adverse effects in aligner therapy. Also, perfect occlusal finishing is immanently complicated by the interposition of aligner material between occluding teeth [39–41]. The results of this study demonstrated that aligners were particularly thick at cusp tips, which constitutes the almost inevitable bite-lowering effect of aligners.

Manual fabrication of aligners inevitably leads to a certain degree of error: manual trimming of the aligner edges causes minor length discrepancies, and manual removal of the aligner from the thermoforming model may lead to shape deformations. Therefore, the thermoforming process was repeated 10-times for each group, and minor differences in thickness were seen at the various measurement locations. However, the quartile ranges were much smaller at the respective measurement points compared to the within-group variability among measurement locations, thus confirming the precise fabrication of aligners in the present investigation. To avoid deformation during micro-CT scanning, the aligners were held in place by polyurethane foam. Nonetheless, minor aligner deformations due to contact to the foam cannot be ruled out.

Despite these minor shortcomings, it could be demonstrated, that micro-CT-scanning is an effective method to assess aligner thickness three-dimensionally. In contrast to previous studies, thickness values were automatically computed upon successful segmentation by means of a 3D-distance transform [42]. This method has the advantage of being resistant against oblique measurements which may occur whenever the micro-CT slices are not orthogonal to aligner surfaces.

Limitations associated with the present analysis include that only upper models were utilized. Due to differences in arch- and tooth-shape, future studies should also investigate thickness homogeneity and the impact of model height for both dental arches. Additionally, only one raw material of the same thickness was utilized. Therefore, it remains unclear whether the results of the present study can be transferred to different aligner polymers and other material thicknesses. Eventually, no a-priori sample size calculation could be performed, as no eligible study could be identified at that time.

In the future, direct 3D-printing of aligners might overcome limitations associated with conventional thermoforming [43]. In 3D-printed aligners, material thickness values may be more homogenous, and unintentional thinning may not occur. Areas of high local stresses may even be specifically thickened to improve stiffness and optimize the resulting force systems.

5. Conclusions

- Micro-CT scanning of aligners followed by automated segmentation and computation material thickness is an eligible approach to analyze material homogeneity
- Manual thermoforming can produce aligners of high repetitious accuracy
- Aligners thermoformed over a higher model exhibited lower material thickness values, especially at facial and palatal surfaces
- Aligners thermoformed over a higher model showed greater homogeneity in material thickness

Author Contributions: B.A.I.: formal analysis, writing—original draft, writing—review & editing. R.K.: investigation, formal analysis, data curation, writing—original draft, writing—review & editing; N.R.: investigation. D.D.: writing—review & editing, supervision. K.B.: conceptualization, investigation, data curation, writing—original draft, writing—review & editing, supervision, project administration. All authors have read and agreed to the published version of the manuscript.

Funding: This research received no external funding.

Institutional Review Board Statement: Not applicable.

Data Availability Statement: Not applicable.

Acknowledgments: The authors express their gratitude to dental technicians Tina Mücke and Axel Dockhorn for their kind help by manufacturing the investigated aligners.

Conflicts of Interest: The authors declare no conflict of interest.

References

1. Q4 and 2018 Corporate Fact Sheet. Available online: http://www.aligntech.com/documents/Align%20Technology%20Corp%20Fact%20Sheet%202018%20Q4.pdf (accessed on 3 March 2021).
2. Ihssen, B.A.; Willmann, J.H.; Nimer, A.; Drescher, D. Effect of in vitro aging by water immersion and thermocycling on the mechanical properties of PETG aligner material. *J. Orofac. Orthop.* **2019**, *80*, 292–303. [CrossRef]
3. Buschang, P.H.; Chastain, D.; Keylor, C.L.; Crosby, D.; Julien, K.C. Incidence of white spot lesions among patients treated with clear aligners and traditional braces. *Angle Orthod.* **2019**, *89*, 359–364. [CrossRef]
4. Rossini, G.; Parrini, S.; Castroflorio, T.; Deregibus, A.; Debernardi, C.L. Periodontal health during clear aligners treatment: A systematic review. *Eur. J. Orthod.* **2015**, *37*, 539–543. [CrossRef]
5. Zhang, B.; Huang, X.-Q.; Huo, S.; Zhang, C.; Zhao, S.; Cen, X.; Zhao, Z. Effect of clear aligners on oral health-related quality of life: A systematic review. *Orthod. Craniofac. Res.* **2020**, *23*, 363–370. [CrossRef] [PubMed]
6. Ke, Y.; Zhu, Y.; Zhu, M. A comparison of treatment effectiveness between clear aligner and fixed appliance therapies. *BMC Oral Health* **2019**, *19*, 24. [CrossRef] [PubMed]
7. Robertson, L.; Kaur, H.; Fagundes, N.C.F.; Romanyk, D.; Major, P.; Mir, C.F. Effectiveness of clear aligner therapy for orthodontic treatment: A systematic review. *Orthod. Craniofac. Res.* **2020**, *23*, 133–142. [CrossRef] [PubMed]
8. Charalampakis, O.; Iliadi, A.; Ueno, H.; Oliver, D.R.; Kim, K.B. Accuracy of clear aligners: A retrospective study of patients who needed refinement. *Am. J. Orthod. Dentofac. Orthop.* **2018**, *154*, 47–54. [CrossRef] [PubMed]
9. Jheon, A.H.; Oberoi, S.; Solem, R.C.; Kapila, S. Moving towards precision orthodontics: An evolving paradigm shift in the planning and delivery of customized orthodontic therapy. *Orthod. Craniofac. Res.* **2017**, *20* (Suppl. 1), 106–113. [CrossRef] [PubMed]
10. Fang, X.; Qi, R.; Liu, C. Root resorption in orthodontic treatment with clear aligners: A systematic review and meta-analysis. *Orthod. Craniofac. Res.* **2019**, *22*, 259–269. [CrossRef] [PubMed]
11. Elhaddaoui, R.; Qoraich, H.S.; Bahije, L.; Zaoui, F. Orthodontic aligners and root resorption: A systematic review. *Int. Orthod.* **2017**, *15*, 1–12. [CrossRef]
12. Gonzales, C.; Hotokezaka, H.; Yoshimatsu, M.; Yozgatian, J.H.; Darendeliler, M.A.; Yoshida, N. Force magnitude and dura-tion effects on amount of tooth movement and root resorption in the rat molar. *Angle Orthod.* **2008**, *78*, 502–509. [CrossRef] [PubMed]
13. Roscoe, M.G.; Meira, J.; Cattaneo, P.M. Association of orthodontic force system and root resorption: A systematic review. *Am. J. Orthod. Dentofac. Orthop.* **2015**, *147*, 610–626. [CrossRef] [PubMed]
14. Elkholy, F.; Panchaphongsaphak, T.; Kilic, F.; Schmidt, F.; Lapatki, B.G. Forces and moments delivered by PET-G aligners to an upper central incisor for labial and palatal translation. *J. Orofac. Orthop.* **2015**, *76*, 460–475. [CrossRef]
15. Elkholy, F.; Schmidt, F.; Jäger, R.; Lapatki, B.G. Forces and moments delivered by novel, thinner PET-G aligners during labiopalatal bodily movement of a maxillary central incisor: An in vitro study. *Angle Orthod.* **2016**, *86*, 883–890. [CrossRef]

16. Hahn, W.; Engelke, B.; Jung, K.; Dathe, H.; Fialka-Fricke, J.; Kubein-Meesenburg, D.; Sadat-Khonsari, R. Initial Forces and Moments Delivered by Removable Thermoplastic Appliances during Rotation of an Upper Central Incisor. *Angle Orthod.* **2010**, *80*, 239–246. [CrossRef]

17. Kohda, N.; Iijima, M.; Muguruma, T.; Brantley, W.A.; Ahluwalia, K.S.; Mizoguchi, I. Effects of mechanical properties of thermoplastic materials on the initial force of thermoplastic appliances. *Angle Orthod.* **2013**, *83*, 476–483. [CrossRef] [PubMed]

18. Hahn, W.; Dathe, H.; Fialka-Fricke, J.; Fricke-Zech, S.; Zapf, A.; Kubein-Meesenburg, D.; Sadat-Khonsari, R. Influence of thermoplastic appliance thickness on the magnitude of force delivered to a maxillary central incisor during tipping. *Am. J. Orthod. Dentofac. Orthop.* **2009**, *136*, 12.e1–12.e7. [CrossRef]

19. Gao, L.; Wichelhaus, A. Forces and moments delivered by the PET-G aligner to a maxillary central incisor for palatal tipping and intrusion. *Angle Orthod.* **2017**, *87*, 534–541. [CrossRef] [PubMed]

20. Jindal, P.; Juneja, M.; Siena, F.L.; Bajaj, D.; Breedon, P. Mechanical and geometric properties of thermoformed and 3D printed clear dental aligners. *Am. J. Orthod. Dentofac. Orthop.* **2019**, *156*, 694–701. [CrossRef]

21. Rüegsegger, P.; Koller, B.; Müller, R. A microtomographic system for the nondestructive evaluation of bone architecture. *Calcif. Tissue Int.* **1996**, *58*, 24–29. [CrossRef]

22. Mantovani, E.; Parrini, S.; Coda, E.; Cugliari, G.; Scotti, N.; Pasqualini, D.; Deregibus, A.; Castroflorio, T. Micro computed tomography evaluation of Invisalign aligner thickness homogeneity. *Angle Orthod.* **2021**, *91*, 343–348. [CrossRef]

23. Lombardo, L.; Palone, M.; Longo, M.; Arveda, N.; Nacucchi, M.; De Pascalis, F.; Spedicato, G.A.; Siciliani, G. MicroCT X-ray comparison of aligner gap and thickness of six brands of aligners: An in-vitro study. *Prog. Orthod.* **2020**, *21*, 12. [CrossRef]

24. Palone, M.; Longo, M.; Arveda, N.; Nacucchi, M.; De Pascalis, F.; Spedicato, G.A.; Siciliani, G.; Lombardo, L. Micro-computed tomography evaluation of general trends in aligner thickness and gap width after thermoforming procedures in-volving six commercial clear aligners: An in vitro study. *Korean J. Orthod.* **2021**, *51*, 135–141. [CrossRef]

25. Hildebrand, T.; Rüegsegger, P. A new method for the model-independent assessment of thickness in three-dimensional images. *J. Microsc.* **1997**, *185*, 67–75. [CrossRef]

26. R Core Team. *R: A Language and Environment for Statistical Computing*; R Foundation for Statistical Computing: Vienna, Austria, 2021.

27. Bates, D.; Mächler, M.; Bolker, B.; Walker, S. Fitting linear mixed-effects models using lme4. *J. Stat. Softw.* **2015**, *67*, 1–48. [CrossRef]

28. Lenth, R.V.; Buerkner, P.; Herve, M.; Love, J.; Riebl, H.; Singmann, H. Estimated Marginal Means, aka Least-Squares Means. Available online: https://cran.r-project.org/web/packages/emmeans/emmeans.pdf (accessed on 10 May 2021).

29. Simon, M.; Keilig, L.; Schwarze, J.; Jung, B.A.; Bourauel, C. Treatment outcome and efficacy of an aligner technique—Regarding incisor torque, premolar derotation and molar distalization. *BMC Oral Health* **2014**, *14*, 68. [CrossRef] [PubMed]

30. Richard, H.A.; Sander, M. *Technische Mechanik. Festigkeitslehre: Lehrbuch mit Praxisbeispielen, Klausuraufgaben und Lösungen*; Vieweg+Teubner: Wiesbaden, Germany, 2008.

31. Jiang, T.; Wu, R.Y.; Wang, J.K.; Wang, H.H.; Tang, G.H. Clear aligners for maxillary anterior en masse retraction: A 3D finite element study. *Sci. Rep.* **2020**, *10*, 1–8. [CrossRef]

32. Rossini, G.; Schiaffino, M.; Parrini, S.; Sedran, A.; Deregibus, A.; Castroflorio, T. Upper Second Molar Distalization with Clear Aligners: A Finite Element Study. *Appl. Sci.* **2020**, *10*, 7739. [CrossRef]

33. Gomez, J.P.; Peña, F.M.; Martínez, V.; Giraldo, D.C.; Cardona, C.I. Initial force systems during bodily tooth movement with plastic aligners and composite attachments: A three-dimensional finite element analysis. *Angle Orthod.* **2015**, *85*, 454–460. [CrossRef] [PubMed]

34. Dasy, H.; Dasy, A.; Asatrian, G.; Rózsa, N.; Lee, H.-F.; Kwak, J.H. Effects of variable attachment shapes and aligner material on aligner retention. *Angle Orthod.* **2015**, *85*, 934–940. [CrossRef] [PubMed]

35. Burstone, C.J.; Choy, K. *The Biomechanical Foundation of Clinical Orthodontics*; Quintessence Publishing Company, Inc.: Chicago, IL, USA, 2015.

36. Krey, K.; Behyar, M.; Hartmann, M.; Corteville, F.; Ratzmann, A. Behaviour of monolayer and multilayer foils in the aligner thermoforming process. *J. Aligner Orthod.* **2019**, *3*, 139–145.

37. Sandhya, V.; Arun, A.; Reddy, V.P.; Mahendra, S.; Chandrashekar, B. Biomechanical Effects of Torquing on Upper Central Incisor with Thermoplastic Aligner: A Comparative Three-Dimensional Finite Element Study with and Without Auxillaries. *J. Indian Orthod. Soc.* **2021**, 1–8. [CrossRef]

38. Wang, J.; Rousso, C.; Christensen, B.I.; Li, P.; Kau, C.H.; MacDougall, M.; Lamani, E. Ethnic differences in the root to crown ratios of the permanent dentition. *Orthod. Craniofac. Res.* **2019**, *22*, 99–104. [CrossRef] [PubMed]

39. Papadimitriou, A.; Mousoulea, S.; Gkantidis, N.; Kloukos, D. Clinical effectiveness of Invisalign® orthodontic treatment: A systematic review. *Prog. Orthod.* **2018**, *19*, 37. [CrossRef] [PubMed]

40. Grünheid, T.; Gaalaas, S.; Hamdan, H.; Larson, B.E. Effect of clear aligner therapy on the buccolingual inclination of mandibular canines and the intercanine distance. *Angle Orthod.* **2016**, *86*, 10–16. [CrossRef] [PubMed]

41. Djeu, G.; Shelton, C.; Maganzini, A. Outcome assessment of Invisalign and traditional orthodontic treatment compared with the American Board of Orthodontics objective grading system. *Am. J. Orthod. Dentofac. Orthop.* **2005**, *128*, 292–298. [CrossRef] [PubMed]

42. Li, J.; Wang, X. A fast 3D euclidean distance transformation. In Proceedings of the 2013 6th International Congress on Image and Signal Processing (CISP), Hangzhou, China, 16–18 December 2013; pp. 875–879.

43. Koenig, N.L. Accuracy of Fit of Direct Printed Aligners versus Thermoformed Aligners. Master's Thesis, Saint Louis University, Saint Louis, MO, USA, 2020.

applied sciences

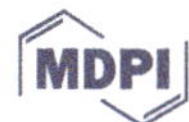

Article

Transfer Accuracy of Two 3D Printed Trays for Indirect Bracket Bonding—An In Vitro Pilot Study

Rebecca Jungbauer [1,*], Jonas Breunig [1], Alois Schmid [2], Mira Hüfner [3], Robert Kerberger [3], Nicole Rauch [4], Peter Proff [1], Dieter Drescher [3] and Kathrin Becker [3]

[1] Department of Orthodontics, University Medical Centre Regensburg, 93053 Regensburg, Germany; jonbreunig@gmail.com (J.B.); Peter.Proff@klinik.uni-regensburg.de (P.P.)
[2] Department of Prosthetic Dentistry, University Medical Centre Regensburg, 93053 Regensburg, Germany; Alois.schmid@ukr.de
[3] Department of Orthodontics, University Hospital Düsseldorf, 40225 Düsseldorf, Germany; mira.huefer@hhu.de (M.H.); Robert.kerberger@med.uni-duesseldorf.de (R.K.); dieter.drescher@med.uni-duesseldorf.de (D.D.); Kathrin.becker@med.uni-duesseldorf.de (K.B.)
[4] Department of Oral Surgery, University Hospital Düsseldorf, 40225 Düsseldorf, Germany; Nicole.rauch@med.uni-duesseldorf.de
[*] Correspondence: Rebecca.jungbauer@klinik.uni-regensburg.de; Tel.: +49-941-16052

Abstract: The present study aimed to investigate the impact of hardness from 3D printed transfer trays and dental crowding on bracket bonding accuracy. Lower models (no crowding group: Little's Irregularity Index (LII) < 3, crowding group: LII > 7, $n = 10$ per group) were selected at random, digitized, 3D printed, and utilized for semiautomated virtual positioning of brackets and tubes. Hard and soft transfer trays were fabricated with polyjet printing and digital light processing, respectively. Brackets and tubes were transferred to the 3D printed models and altogether digitized using intraoral scanning (IOS) and microcomputed tomography (micro-CT) for assessment of linear and angular deviations. Mean intra- and interrater reliability amounted to $0.67 \pm 0.34 / 0.79 \pm 0.16$ for IOS, and $0.92 \pm 0.05 / 0.92 \pm 0.5$ for the micro-CT measurements. Minor linear discrepancies were observed (median: 0.11 mm, Q1–Q3: −0.06–0.28 mm). Deviations in torque (median: 2.49°, Q1–Q3: 1.27–4.03°) were greater than angular ones (median: 1.81°, Q1–Q3: 1.05°–2.90°), higher for hard (median: 2.49°, Q1–Q3: 1.32–3.91°) compared to soft (median: 1.77°, Q1–Q3: 0.94–3.01°) trays ($p < 0.001$), and torque errors were more pronounced at crowded front teeth ($p < 0.05$). In conclusion, the clinician should carefully consider the potential impact of hardness and crowding on bracket transfer accuracy, specifically in torque and angular orientation.

Keywords: bonding tray; 3D-printing; intraoral scanning; shore hardness

Citation: Jungbauer, R.; Breunig, J.; Schmid, A.; Hüfner, M.; Kerberger, R.; Rauch, N.; Proff, P.; Drescher, D.; Becker, K. Transfer Accuracy of Two 3D Printed Trays for Indirect Bracket Bonding—An In Vitro Pilot Study. *Appl. Sci.* **2021**, *11*, 6013. https://doi.org/10.3390/app11136013

Academic Editor: Dorina Lauritano

Received: 11 June 2021
Accepted: 25 June 2021
Published: 28 June 2021

Publisher's Note: MDPI stays neutral with regard to jurisdictional claims in published maps and institutional affiliations.

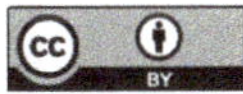

1. Introduction

For orthodontic treatment of malocclusions, the insertion of fixed multibracket appliances is a common and reliable treatment option. Since the introduction of the straight-wire technique, ideal positioning of bracket has become of eminent importance [1–5]. Incorrectly positioned brackets can lead to undesirable tooth movement and extended treatment time.

Instead of chairside positioning (direct bonding), ideal bracket positions can be planned prior to treatment (indirect bonding). This approach was first described by Silverman and Cohen in 1972 [6] and has the advantage of unrestricted vision, reduced chair time, and increased patient comfort [7]. With regard to the rate of bracket loss in vivo and shear bond strength in vitro, direct and indirect approaches were reported to be comparable [8–11]. In the classical indirect bonding technique, brackets are positioned on plaster models and transfer templates are fabricated in the laboratory [12,13], which are frequently made of single- or double-layer silicones, vacuum-formed sheets of various thicknesses or a combination of both [14–18]. Nowadays, computer-assisted processes offer a time efficient alternative. Software tools allow for semiautomated determination of ideal bracket positions and virtual design of transfer trays [19], which are commonly manufactured by means of 3D printing.

Few in vitro studies compared transfer accuracy of CAD/CAM technology for indirect bracket placement to conventional ones and revealed comparable accuracies [20–22]. However, it is not yet clear whether severe crowding and the hardness of 3D-printed transfer trays impact on bracket transfer accuracy. Additionally, the workflow to assess potential bracket transfer inaccuracies remains to be validated, as artefacts from intraoral scanning may impair the measurements [23].

Therefore, the present study aimed at investigating the impact of transfer tray hardness and crowding on bracket transfer accuracy, and to validate whether intraoral scanning is an eligible tool to assess potential errors.

2. Materials and Methods

2.1. Selection of Casts

Twenty pre-treatment plaster models from the lower jaw were selected at random from the archive of the Department of Orthodontics, University Medical Centre Regensburg such that $n = 10$ models exhibited minor crowding (Little's Irregularity Index (LII) < 3, "no crowding" group), and another $n = 10$ showed severe crowding (LII > 7, "crowding group"). The classification was performed with a digital caliper according to the LII, as described previously [24].

The following exclusion criteria were applied: no permanent dentition or second molars not completely erupted, agenesis, previous extractions, dental anomalies, displaced or retained canines, patients with syndromes. The study workflow is provided in detail in Figure 1.

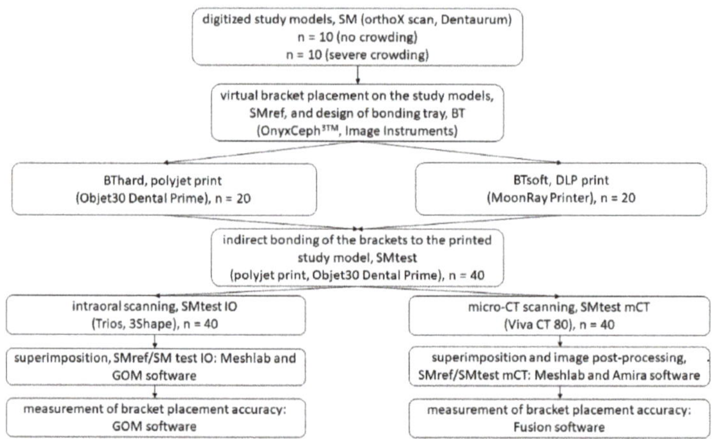

Figure 1. Flow diagram detailing the study workflow.

2.2. Model Preparation and Bracket Placement

The original plaster models were digitized using a 3D model scanner (orthoX®scan, Dentaurum, Ispringen, Germany). Each of the generated digital study models (SM) was printed twice using the Objet30 Dental Prime printer (Stratasys, Eden Prairie, MN, USA) using the high-speed mode (28 micron), VeroGlaze MED620 material and SUP705 support material (both Stratasys, Eden Prairie, MN, USA). The models were cleaned with a water jet and served as study models to which the brackets were bonded later (Figure 2A,B). Until usage they were stored in dry rice as reported previously and recommended by the manufacturer [25].

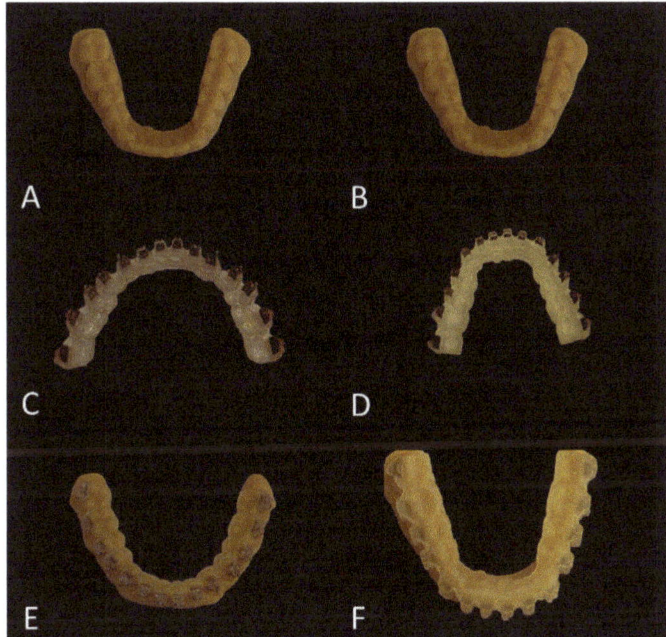

Figure 2. Overview of the bracket placement workflow. (**A,B**) Printed study models (SM). (**C,D**) Hard (**C**) and soft (**D**) tray with brackets placed inside the respective molds. (**E,F**) Printed casts with the brackets indirectly bonded by means of the hard (**E**) and soft (**F**) transfer tray.

The SM were imported into a proprietary software (OnyxCeph^{3TM} Lab software, Image Instruments, Chemnitz, Germany) for virtual placement of brackets/tubes utilizing the FA-Bonding module as follows: teeth 35–45 (Discovery smart bracket, Dentaurum, Ispringen, Germany), teeth 36, 37, 46, 47 (Ortho-Cast M series buccal tubes, Dentaurum, Ispringen, Germany).

The FA-Bonding module operates semiautomatically and utilizes the facial axis (FA) for automated bracket positioning along the vertical tooth axis. Minor adjustments were performed by one single experienced orthodontist (RJ). The SM together with the virtually placed brackets served as reference models (SMref) (Figure 3).

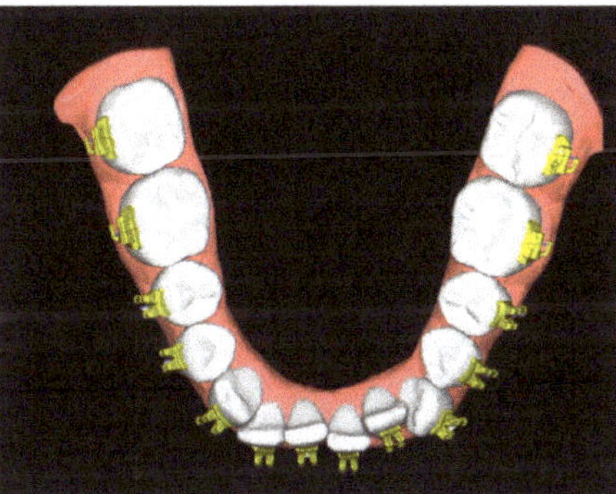

Figure 3. Reference model consisting of a digitized study model and the semiautomatically positioned brackets/tubes (SMref).

2.3. Planning and Printing of the Transfer Trays

The transfer trays were designed using the Bonding Tray 3D module (OnyxCeph[3TM] Lab software). A base covering the teeth and molds for the brackets and tubes was designed. In detail, the base had a thickness of 1 mm and covered all the occlusal/incisal surfaces as well as half of the lingual and about 1/3 of the labial surfaces of every tooth. The molds had a 0.6 mm thickness and covered the occlusal part of the brackets/tubes and overlapped the slot by 0.04 mm. Undercutting parts (up to 0.5 mm) were filled by the software.

Each tray was printed twice, one time with a hard and another with a soft printing material (Figure 2C,D): the hard transfer trays were printed horizontally in a polyjet printing process (Objet30 Dental Prime, Stratasys, Eden Prairie, MN, USA) using the high-speed mode (28 micron resolution) and biocompatible MED610 (shore D hardness 83–86; Stratasys, Eden Prairie, MN, USA) with support material SUP705 (Stratasys, Eden Prairie, MN, USA). After printing, the support material was removed by water jet cleaning and a hard toothbrush. The soft transfer trays were printed horizontally by means of a digital light processing (DLP) using the MoonRay Printer (SprintRay, LA, USA) with a 100 micron resolution and the biocompatible NextDent Ortho IBT (shore A 85 hardness; NextDent B.V., Soesterberg, The Netherlands).

After printing, the trays were washed for 20 min with Isopropanol (FormWash, Form-labs, Berlin, Germany) and light cured for 60 min at 45 °C (Curebox, Wicked Engineering, East Windsor, NJ, USA). For those trays that were printed with the DLP technology, an occlusal overlay plane was designed to avoid the need of adding support structures and increase the adhesion to the platform as it became possible to locate them horizontally.

2.4. Bracket Transfer and Bonding

For both types of transfer trays (hard and soft), the brackets and tubes were carefully positioned inside the respective molds (Figure 2C,D). A thin layer of dental wax was placed between the tubes and the tray to enable stable fixation. Then, the facial bases of the brackets and tubes were cleaned with acetone, and a thin layer of TransbondXT adhesive (3M, Monrovia, CA, USA) was applied to the bracket's base and homogenously dispersed with a microbrush and a thin layer of TransbondXT primer (3M, Monrovia, CA, USA).

The templates were placed on the study models (Figure 2E,F) and gently fixated manually during curing with the Ortholux Luminous Curing Light (1600 mW/cm^2, 3M, Monrovia, CA, USA). Curing was performed at each bracket and tube for 6 s at the mesial and distal site, respectively. Afterwards, the transfer trays were carefully removed, and excessive resin was eliminated using a frontal sickle scaler (HuFriedy, Frankfurt am Main, Germany) and adhesive removers at 10.000 rpm (Komet Dental, Lemgo, Germany). Until digitization, all study models with the bonded brackets and tubes (SMtest) were stored in boxes filled with dry rice [25].

2.5. Digitization, Image Processing and Measurement of Bracket Placement Accuracy
2.5.1. Intraoral Scanning

SMtest models were covered with a thin layer of scanning spray (BlueSpray, Dreve Dentamid, Unna, Germany). The as-prepared models were digitized using an intraoral scanner (Trios 3, 3Shape, Kopenhagen, Denmark; setting: typical clinical setting, full arch scanning mode). Image registration of the SMtest-IO with SMref was achieved in two steps: first, a reference-point based pre-alignment was performed in MeshLab (MeshLab v1.3.3, Visual Computing Lab, ISTI, CNR). Fine registration was realized using the local best fit algorithm implemented in GOM Inspect 2018 software (GOM, Braunschweig, Germany). The fine-registration procedure was repeated until convergence as described earlier [26].

To assess the 3D accuracy of bracket placement, surface comparison was utilized. In case intraorally scanned brackets showed scanning errors (Figure 4B,C), the most likely correct areas were identified by a trained observer, which led to exclusion of the hooks at all brackets and tubes (Figure 4A). The minimum, maximum, mean and standard deviation values between SMtest-IO and SMref were recorded for each bracket and tube.

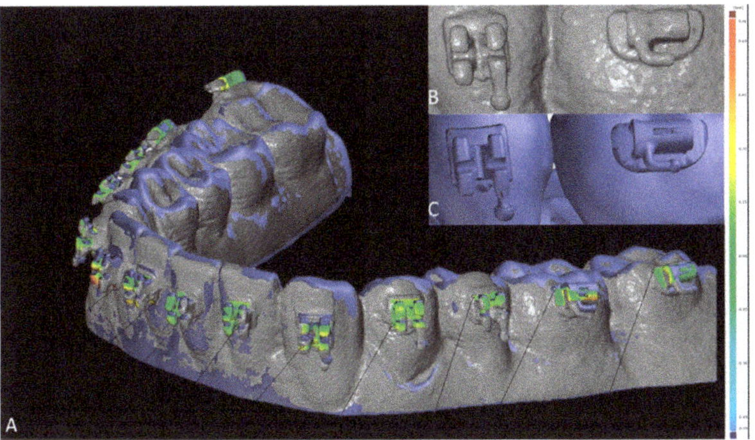

Figure 4. Measurement of the bracket transfer accuracy with GOM software. (**A**) Superimposed study models scanned with intraoral scanner (SMtest-IO) visualized in grey and reference study models (SMref) visualized in blue; distances are coded by heatmap coloring. (**B**) Scanned brackets from SMtest-IO in higher magnification. (**C**) Original brackets from SMref in higher magnification.

2.5.2. Micro-CT Scanning (Method Validation)

Digitization of SMtest was also achieved using a micro-CT (Viva CT 80, Scanco Medical, Brüttisellen, Switzerland). The scans were performed at 70 kVp, 114 µA, 535 ms integration time and 2× frame averaging, and reconstructed to a nominal isotropic voxel size of 39 µm. The so achieved SMtest-mCT models were segmented and surfaces were extracted using Amira software (v2019, Thermo Fisher Scientific, Berlin, Germany).

SMtest-mCT surfaces were aligned with the respective SMref models using a landmark-based registration procedure followed by an iterative closest point algorithm (Meshlab software) as described earlier [26]. Owing to metal artefacts on the micro-CT scans, each scanned bracket on the SMtest was replaced with the respective original bracket surface by superimposing the latter on the micro-scanned ones (Amira software). This technique enabled preservation of the true positions of the brackets on the digitized SMtest models (Figure 5A,B).

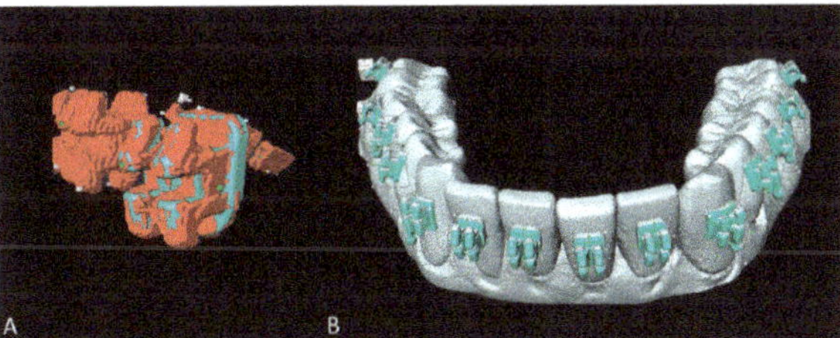

Figure 5. Superimposition and image post-processing with Amira software. (**A**) Micro-CT scanned brackets (red) and the superimposed original brackets (green). (**B**) Reference study models (SMref) visualized in grey and corrected brackets from micro-CT scanned study models (SMtest-mCT) visualized in turquoise.

Bracket placement accuracy on SMtest-mCT models was assessed using Fusion 360 (Autodesk, San Rafael, CA, USA). All brackets and tubes were virtually separated from SMref and oriented along the global Cartesian coordinate system, and an additional local coordinate system was defined for every bracket/tube (Figure 6A). The disagreement between brackets from SMtest-mCT and SMref along the x-, y- and z-axes was recorded as mesial/distal, occlusal/gingival, buccal/oral deviation. The angular deviation between the vertical bracket axes was recorded as torque, and between the horizontal axes as angulation discrepancy (Figure 6B).

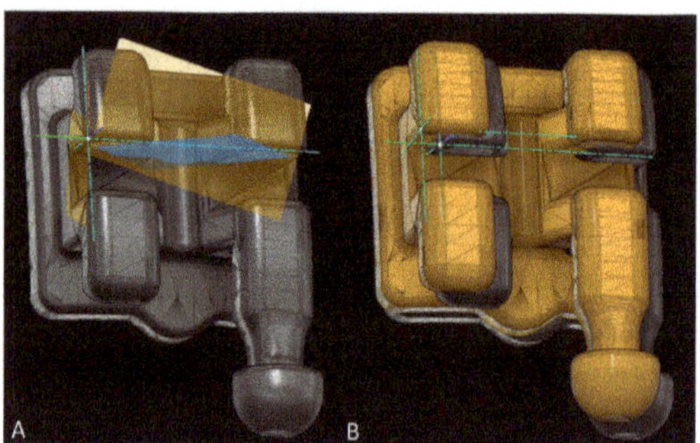

Figure 6. Measurement of bracket transfer accuracy with Fusion software; (**A**) reference bracket with the local coordinate system defined through the three planes (yellow and blue). (**B**) Reference bracket and test bracket (yellow) to measure the linear and angular bracket bonding accuracy (mm, degree).

2.6. Sample Size Calculation

According to Pottier et al. [21] 91 observations per group would be necessary to detect a moderate effect size at a significance level of 0.05 with a 90% power. Therefore, 10 study models were included in each group.

2.7. Reliability of Measurements

To calculate intra- and interrater reliability, 20 casts were selected at random and all measurements, including the matching process, were performed again by the same investigator after a time interval of 4 weeks, and also by a second experienced investigator. To calculate the systematic error, the intraclass correlation coefficient (ICC; two-way mixed, absolute agreement) was calculated.

2.8. Statistical Analysis

The software IBM SPSS Statistics 25 (IBM, Armonk, NY, USA) and R [27] were used to analyze the data. For descriptive purposes, boxplots were created. According to *Kolmogorov–Smirnov* tests and visual inspection of boxplots, not all the data showed normal distribution. Thus, non-parametric *Mann–Whitney* U-test was used to compare brackets/tubes placed at casts with/without crowding, as well as for brackets/tubes bonded with hard/soft trays for linear and angular measurements at the molars, premolars, canines and incisors, respectively. The effect size r was calculated and interpreted in accordance with *Cohen* likewise to *Pearson* r, i.e., <0.3: low effect size; 0.3–0.5: medium effect size; >0.5: good effect size) [28].

3. Results

3.1. Reliability of Measurements

When SMtest-mCT models were utilized, the workflow reliability ranged from high to excellent. In detail, mean intra- and interrater reliability amounted to 0.917 ± 0.053 and 0.921 ± 0.045, respectively (Table S1 in Supplementary Materials). Visual inspection confirmed that artefact-impaired brackets from micro-CT scanning could be substituted with artefact-free surfaces from the original brackets by means of surface alignment, thus enabling accurate measurements of the metric and angular deviations.

When SMtest-IO models were utilized, mean intra- and interrater reliability amounted to 0.674 ± 0.341 and 0.785 ± 0.161, respectively, and ranged from -0.073 to 0.979 for intrarater, and from 0.388 to 0.975 for interrater values. A total of 12.5% (intrarater) and 31.3% (interrater) of the measurements indicated moderate reliability (ICC 0.50–0.75) and

25% (intrarater) as well as 6.3% (interrater) of the values demonstrated poor reliability (ICC < 0.5), respectively (Table S1 in Supplementary Materials). The low reliabilities owed to the fact that bracket surfaces digitized with the intraoral scanner presented several artefacts, which impaired identification of reliable areas to assess bracket transfer accuracy. Therefore, the SMtest-IO models were excluded at this point from the study, and only bracket transfer deviations assessed with the SMtest-mCT were reported.

3.2. Bracket Bonding Accuracy (Linear Measurements)

Boxplots of linear measurements are provided in Figure 7. Discrepancies were most pronounced in the buccal/oral (median: 0.18 mm, Q1–Q3: 0.06–0.30 mm) compared to the mesial/distal (median: 0.054 mm, Q1–Q3: −0.18–0.26 mm) and occlusal/gingival direction (median: 0.06 mm, Q1– Q3: −0.11–0.23 mm). Linear discrepancies were more present at incisors (median: 0.15 mm, Q1–Q3: −0.02–0.31 mm) and canines (median: 0.16 mm, Q1–Q3: 0.01–0.23 mm) compared to molars (median: 0.05 mm, Q1–Q3: −0.01–0.21 mm) and premolars (median: 0.10 mm, Q1–Q3: −0.07–0.25 mm).

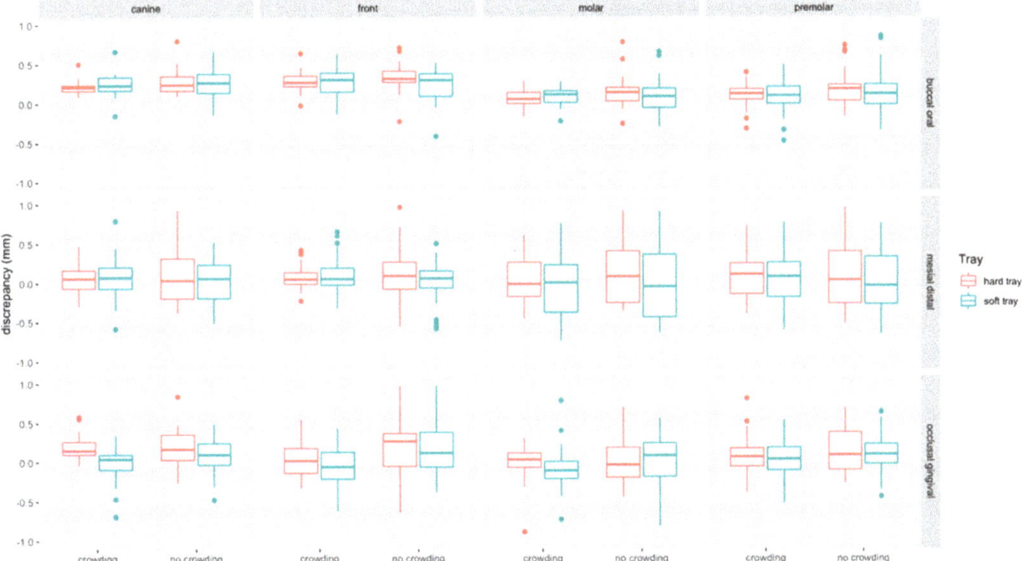

Figure 7. Boxplots detailing the accuracy of bracket transfer for lingual measurements. Results are summarized for the canines, front teeth, molars, and premolars and split up into hard/soft trays and no crowding/crowding. A positive/negative value indicates mesial/distal, buccal/oral or occlusal/gingival displacement, respectively.

3.2.1. Impact of Crowding

Linear discrepancies were higher in the no crowding (median: 0.14 mm, Q1–Q3: −0.06–0.30 mm) compared to the crowding (median: 0.10 mm, Q1–Q3: −0.06–0.23 mm) group ($p < 0.001$). When splitting the data to assess the impact of crowding for the two types of trays and the respective tooth types, significant differences were found in occlusal/gingival direction, i.e., for hard and soft trays at front teeth ($p = 0.015$, $p = 0.001$, respectively), and for soft trays in the molar region ($p = 0.007$). For hard trays, a significant difference was noted in buccal-oral direction at molars ($p = 0.029$) (Table 1).

Table 1. Descriptive statistics for the subgroup analysis of the bracket transfer accuracies for linear and angular measurements. Results are summarized for the canines, front teeth, molars, and premolars and split up into hard/soft trays and no crowding/crowding. A positive/negative value indicates mesial/distal, buccal/oral or occlusal/gingival displacement. Medians (MD) and interquartile ranges (IQR), mm or degree are given. Comparison between crowding vs. no crowding groups and hard vs. soft trays was performed using the *Mann–Whitney* U-test. The *p*-values for comparison of hard vs. soft trays are presented in the lines, for crowding vs. no crowding in the right column. *Pearson*-correlation coefficient (r) was calculated in addition to measure the effect size, and was interpreted as follows: <0.3 low, 0.3–0.5 medium, >0.5 good effect size.

Tooth Type	Tray	Measurement	MD	IQR	MD	IQR	*p*-Value
			No crowding (LII < 3)		Crowding (LII > 7)		Crowding vs. no crowding
	Hard	Angulation (°)	4.02	1.33	5.07	2.88	0.529
	Soft	Angulation (°)	1.86	2.07	2.04	2.59	0.445
	p-value hard vs. soft tray (r)		<0.001 (0.58) ***		<0.001 (0.56) ***		
	Hard	Buccal/oral (mm)	0.24	0.2	0.21	0.09	0.201
	Soft	Buccal/oral (mm)	0.27	0.29	0.23	0.18	0.698
	p-value hard vs. soft tray (r)		0.968		0.327		
Canine (*n* = 40)	Hard	Mesial/distal (mm)	0.04	0.54	0.06	0.24	0.989
	Soft	Mesial/distal (mm)	0.06	0.45	0.07	0.38	0.678
	p-value hard vs. soft tray (r)		0.495		0.841		
	Hard	Occlusal/gingival (mm)	0.16	0.37	0.15	0.24	0.799
	Soft	Occlusal/gingival (mm)	0.10	0.29	0.04	0.21	0.211
	p-value hard vs. soft tray (r)		0.398		0.005 (0.45) **		
	Hard	Torque (°)	4.32	2.63	4.7	3.32	0.461
	Soft	Torque (°)	3.52	3.04	2.51	5.04	0.341
	p-value hard vs. soft tray. (r)		0.289		0.096		
	Hard	Angulation (°)	1.96	1.7	2.46	2.25	0.053
	Soft	Angulation (°)	1.59	1.19	1.29	1.64	0.178
	p-value hard vs. soft tray (r)		0.308		0.001 (0.39) **		
	Hard	Buccal/oral (mm)	0.32	0.15	0.27	0.14	0.083
	Soft	Buccal/oral (mm)	0.30	0.30	0.3	0.24	0.722
	p-value hard vs. soft tray (r)		0.065		0.923		
Front (*n* = 80)	Hard	Mesial/distal (mm)	0.09	0.38	0.05	0.15	0.607
	Soft	Mesial/distal (mm)	0.06	0.22	0.05	0.26	0.624
	p-value hard vs. soft tray (r)		0.384		0.769		
	Hard	Occlusal/gingival (mm)	0.26	0.43	0.02	0.32	0.015 (0.27) *
	Soft	Occlusal/gingival (mm)	0.12	0.45	−0.07	0.37	0.001 (0.36) *
	p-value hard vs. soft tray (r)		0.554		0.068		
	Hard	Torque (°)	2.31	2.01	3.28	2.49	0.028 (0.25) *
	Soft	Torque (°)	1.64	2.34	1.54	2.07	0.439
	p-value hard vs. soft tray (r)		0.312		<0.001 (0.41) ***		

Table 1. *Cont.*

Tooth Type	Tray	Measurement	MD	IQR	MD	IQR	*p*-Value
	Hard	Angulation (°)	2.11	2.01	1.73	1.22	0.163
	Soft	Angulation (°)	1.8	1.35	1.65	2.8	0.577
	p-value hard vs. soft tray (r)		0.366		0.773		
	Hard	Buccal/oral (mm)	0.14	0.17	0.06	0.15	0.029 (0.24) *
	Soft	Buccal/oral (mm)	0.10	0.25	0.12	0.15	0.6
	p-value hard vs. soft tray (r)		0.14		0.296		
Molar	Hard	Mesial/distal (mm)	0.08	0.68	−0.01	0.45	0.788
(*n* = 80)	Soft	Mesial/distal (mm)	−0.04	0.82	0.07	0.66	0.893
	p-value (hard vs. soft tray)		0.159		0.368		
	Hard	Occlusal/gingival (mm)	−0.03	0.4	0.03	0.22	0.61
	Soft	Occlusal/gingival (mm)	0.09	0.43	−0.12	0.23	0.007 (0.30) **
	p-value hard vs. soft tray (r)		0.583		0.002 (0.34) **		
	Hard	Torque (°)	3.61	4.73	2.71	3.04	0.405
	Soft	Torque (°)	2.26	2.23	3.23	5.27	0.470
	p-value hard vs. soft tray (r)		0.189		0.7		
	Hard	Angulation (°)	1.59	1.7	1.79	1.66	0.707
	Soft	Angulation (°)	1.43	1.63	1.3	1.11	0.178
	p-value hard vs. soft tray (r)		0.441		0.009 (0.29) **		
	Hard	Buccal/oral (mm)	0.19	0.23	0.13	0.14	0.119
	Soft	Buccal/oral (mm)	0.14	0.29	0.10	0.22	0.56
	p-value hard vs. soft tray (r)		0.242		0.14		
Premolar	Hard	Mesial/distal (mm)	0.04	0.67	0.11	0.41	0.9
(*n* = 80)	Soft	Mesial/distal (mm)	−0.03	0.61	0.12	0.5	0.669
	p-value hard vs. soft tray (r)		0.634		0.954		
	Hard	Occlusal/gingival (mm)	0.09	0.54	0.07	0.29	0.462
	Soft	Occlusal/gingival (mm)	0.1	0.28	0.04	0.29	0.248
	p-value hard vs. soft tray (r)		0.747		0.488		
	Hard	Torque (°)	2.60	2.03	2.46	1.94	0.476
	Soft	Torque (°)	1.96	1.83	2.05	2.03	0.693
	p-value hard vs. soft tray (r)		0.057		0.163		

$* p < 0.05 ** p < 0.01. *** p < 0.001.$

3.2.2. Impact of Tray Type

Linear discrepancies were higher for hard (median: 0.13 mm, Q1–Q3: −0.05–0.27 mm) compared to the soft (median: −0.08 mm, Q1–Q3: −0.08–0.26 mm) trays ($p = 0.004$). When splitting the data, significant differences were only detected in occlusal/gingival direction within the crowding group, i.e., at canines ($p = 0.005$), where the soft tray performed more accurately, and at molars ($p = 0.002$), where the soft trays transferred the tubes more gingivally (Table 1).

3.3. Bracket Bonding Accuracy (Angular Measurements)

The boxplots of angular measurements are provided in Figure 8. Discrepancies in torque (median: 2.49°, Q1–Q3: 1.27–4.03°) were higher than in angulation (median: 1.81°, Q1–Q3: 1.05–2.90°). Discrepancies were most pronounced at canines (median: 3.50°, Q1–Q3: −1.81–5.15°) and comparable at front teeth (median: 1.96°, Q1–Q3: 1.01–3.02 mm), molars (median: 2.09°, Q1–Q3: 1.09–3.79°) and premolars (median: 1.82°, Q1–Q3: 1.05–2.90°).

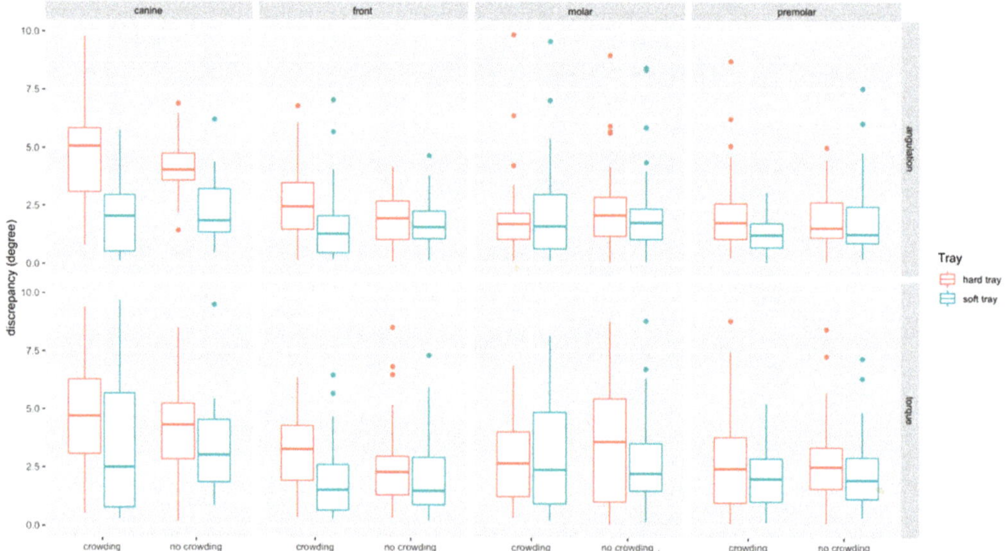

Figure 8. Boxplots detailing the accuracy of bracket transfer for angular measurements. Results are summarized for the canines, front teeth, molars, and premolars and split up into hard/soft trays and no crowding/crowding.

3.3.1. Impact of Crowding

Angular discrepancies were by trend higher in the crowding (median: 2.16°, Q1–Q3: 1.21–3.67°) compared to the no-crowding (median: 2.08°, Q1–Q3: 1.01–2.7°) group ($p = 0.358$). When splitting the data to assess the impact of crowding for the two types of trays and the respective tooth types, significant differences were found for torque at hard trays in the front region ($p = 0.028$) (Table 1).

3.3.2. Impact of the Tray Type

Angular discrepancies were higher for hard (median: 2.49°, Q1–Q3: 1.32–3.91°) compared to the soft (median: 1.77°, Q1–Q3: 0.94–3.01°) trays ($p < 0.001$). When splitting the data, significant differences were found in the crowding group, i.e., for angulation at front teeth ($p = 0.001$), canines ($p < 0.001$) and premolars ($p = 0.009$), and for torque at front teeth ($p < 0.001$), and in the no crowding group for angulation at canines ($p < 0.001$). For all these differences the transfer with the soft tray was more accurate (Table 1).

4. Discussion

The aim of the present in vitro study was to assess whether the hardness (shore A 85 vs. shore D83 –86) of 3D printed transfer trays and severe crowding impact on bracket bonding accuracy. Additionally, it was aimed to validate the workflow.

In the literature, different procedures for digitizing study models, e.g., intraoral scanners, 3D-model scanners or cone beam computed tomography (CBCT), were described for assessing the accuracy of transfer trays in digital workflows [29–32]. Matching intraoral scans (IOS) with the virtually planned reference models seems to be used most frequently and has the advantage that this workflow can be easily applied to clinical as well as in vitro settings, whereas microcomputed tomography (micro-CT) is limited to in vitro studies only. Nevertheless, full arch scanning in the presence of brackets might have an impact on scanning accuracy [33,34] and could therefore affect outcomes achieved with this technology. Previous studies did not evaluate the accuracy of workflows for assessing the accuracy of transfer trays or did not indicate whether the whole process including image registration was repeated to assess reliability. In our study, ICC values for intraorally scanned models indicated a very low reliability likely owing to significant artifacts at the scanned metal brackets and tubes. To some extent scanning accuracy may be impeded by the thin layer of scanning powder applied to the brackets, as scanning powder is suspected to increase scanning errors [35]. Nonetheless, distortion of the bracket area in intraoral scans was reported recently [36]. In the present analysis, the references and scanned surfaces showed a visible incongruence. Although only the apparently matching regions from the brackets were utilized for comparison in GOM software as described in [29], the intra- and interrater reliability ranged from excellent to poor in our experiment. Therefore, and despite having been used in the majority of previous experiments, the IOS approach was not found eligible to assess the accuracy of transfer trays in the present investigation. Instead, micro-CT scanning proved to be a highly reliable approach. Therefore, only the deviation measurements performed with this approach were reported.

The micro-CT workflow revealed minor linear discrepancies between planned and achieved bracket positions ranging from −0.06 to 0.28 mm (1st–3rd quartile). Interestingly, linear deviations were slightly but significantly lower in severe crowding situations, whereas no overall impact of crowding was identified. In the subgroup analysis, significant differences were most frequently observed at front teeth, where brackets were bonded more accurately in occlusal/gingival direction when severe crowding was present. In contrast, in crowding groups, tubes were located significantly more gingival when soft trays were utilized.

Angular deviations were by trend higher when crowding was present, and torque discrepancies reached significance at front teeth. Bracket transfer with hard trays resulted in greater angular deviations compared to soft trays. The greatest impact of bracket hardness was noted on canines, where soft trays improved median angular discrepancies by 2.16° and 3.03° in no crowding and crowding situations, respectively.

Regarding the amount of deviations, linear discrepancies ≤ 0.5 mm and angular deviations of $\leq 2°$ were considered to be acceptable as suggested by The American Board of Orthodontists (ABO) [37] and further studies [21,32], despite some authors recommending more strict ranges [30,38].

In the present analysis, linear discrepancies were within the ABO range of 0.5 mm, which is also in line with previous findings [20,21,29]. Deviations in torque were greater than in angulation. Especially when brackets were bonded with hard trays, values were frequently greater than 2° and also clearly higher as reported previously [20,21,29]. Besides the digitization method and measurement workflow, reasons for the greater angular deviations may also owe to the design of the trays, handling, crowding, and material properties, as discussed below.

Few studies investigated the transfer accuracy of 3D printed transfer trays. Zhang et al. compared different variants (3D printed trays for each single tooth versus 3D printed trays for the whole dental arch) with two types of double-layer vacuum formed trays and found no significant differences [22]). However, this study performed caliper measurements in a single direction only. Niu et al. found that 3D printed trays provided better transfer accuracy compared to vacuum-formed ones, and in line with the present investigation, linear control was superior to angular control, whereas angular values also exceeded the ABO-ranges [20]. In contrast, satisfactory angular control was reported for an L-type design of 3D printed trays that was employed in an in vivo study by Xue et al. {29}. This approach is of particular interest, as it provided a positioning template. This allowed a combination of direct bonding and a-priori planning of bracket positions. When comparing 3D printed with conventional silicone trays, Pottier et al. reported that conventional silicone enabled a more accurate bracket transfer [24], and accurate bracket transfer using silicone trays was also reported by other authors [18,38]. The high precision of this conventional laboratory workflow may owe to the material properties of silicone. Additionally, brackets are fully covered by the tray which may prevent bracket movement during transfer.

In contrast, due to material properties of the 3D printed transfer trays, no full coverage of brackets was possible, and the trays overlapped the slots by 0.04 mm only. This design resulted in a difficult handling specifically at front teeth and canines in the presence of crowding because brackets were located remarkably close to each other. Additionally, placement in hard trays was particularly challenging as brackets had to be pressed with the fingertips into the tight molds. Whereas bracket placement was easier in the soft tray group, brackets did not remain stable in their position when minor deformations of the soft tray occurred. This might explain the more gingival placement of molar tubes in the presence of severe crowding.

To the best knowledge of the authors, no previous study investigated the impact of crowding and hardness of the bonding tray on bracket transfer accuracy. Against our a-priori assumptions, linear bracket transfer accuracy was slightly but significantly higher in the crowding group. Interestingly, crowded front teeth seemed to improve the vertical fit of the trays, thus prohibiting a gingival bracket displacement. However, when hard transfers were utilized the tight fit of the transfer tray did not prevent deviations in torque, which were most pronounced at front teeth and canines in the present of crowding. The authors suspect that this might be explained by increased tension due to severely crowded incisors resulting in deformation of the lower part of the hard tray. In the presence of crowding bonding with the hard tray further resulted in increased angular deviations at front teeth, canines and premolars.

One of limitations of the present study is that cases with mild crowding (LII 3–7) were not included since the present study aimed at assessing whether crowding has an overall impact. The fact that the present study reports in vitro findings, and that the micro-CT workflow cannot be established for clinical trials, needs to be considered as another limitation. Additionally, the present study did not evaluate different designs in terms of thickness, extension and bracket covering, and further materials. Eventually, the impact of the different resolutions of the two printing technologies could not be assessed.

5. Conclusions

- The present study found that intraoral scanning may severely impede measurements to assess the accuracy of bracket transfer, whereas micro-CT was shown to be a highly reliable alternative for in vitro settings.
- We demonstrated that linear discrepancies were below the ABO-range of 0.5 mm, most of the angular discrepancies were not within the clinical acceptable limit of $2°$.
- Severe crowding and transfer tray hardness have an impact on transfer tray accuracy, and bonding with the soft transfer tray was more accurate in cases of severe crowding.
- Front teeth were most frequently affected by bonding errors, followed by canines and molars.

Supplementary Materials: The following are available online at https://www.mdpi.com/article/10.3390/app11136013/s1. Table S1: Intra- and interrater reliability of the different workflows.

Author Contributions: R.J.: Conceptualization, methodology, investigation, formal analysis, writing—original draft. J.B.: investigation, writing—review and editing. A.S.: methodology, investigation, writing—review and editing. M.H.: investigation, writing—review and editing. R.K.: investigation, writing—review and editing. N.R.: investigation, writing—review and editing. P.P.: resources, supervision, writing—review and editing. D.D.: resources, supervision, writing—review and editing. K.B.: conceptualization, investigation, formal analysis, writing—original draft. All authors have read and agreed to the published version of the manuscript.

Funding: This research received no external funding.

Institutional Review Board Statement: Not applicable.

Informed Consent Statement: Not applicable.

Data Availability Statement: Data will be provided upon reasonable request.

Acknowledgments: The authors thank Dentaurum and C3D.digital for donating the brackets/tubes and the DLP printed transfer trays utilized in the present investigation.

Conflicts of Interest: All authors declare no conflict of interest.

References

1. Andrews, L.F. The six keys to normal occlusion. *Am. J. Orthod.* **1972**, *62*, 296–309. [CrossRef]
2. Andrews, L.F. The straight-wire appliance, origin, controversy, commentary. *J. Clin. Orthod.* **1976**, *10*, 99–114.
3. Andrews, L.F. The straight-wire appliance. Explained and compared. *J. Clin. Orthod.* **1976**, *10*, 174–195. [PubMed]
4. Andrews, L.F. *Straight Wire: The Concept and Appliance*; Wells: San Diego, CA, USA, 1989; ISBN 0961625600.
5. Shpack, N.; Geron, S.; Floris, I.; Davidovitch, M.; Brosh, T.; Vardimon, A.D. Bracket placement in lingual vs labial systems and direct vs indirect bonding. *Angle Orthod.* **2007**, *77*, 509–517. [CrossRef]
6. Silverman, E.; Cohen, M.; Gianelly, A.A.; Dietz, V.S. A universal direct bonding system for both metal and plastic brackets. *Am. J. Orthod.* **1972**, *62*, 236–244. [CrossRef]
7. Sondhi, A. Efficient and effective indirect bonding. *Am. J. Orthod. Dentofac. Orthop.* **1999**, *115*, 352–359. [CrossRef]
8. Yi, G.K.; Dunn, W.J.; Taloumis, L.J. Shear bond strength comparison between direct and indirect bonded orthodontic brackets. *Am. J. Orthod. Dentofac. Orthop.* **2003**, *124*, 577–581. [CrossRef]
9. Linn, B.J.; Berzins, D.W.; Dhuru, V.B.; Bradley, T.G. A comparison of bond strength between direct- and indirect-bonding methods. *Angle Orthod.* **2006**, *76*, 289–294. [CrossRef]
10. Menini, A.; Cozzani, M.; Sfondrini, M.F.; Scribante, A.; Cozzani, P.; Gandini, P. A 15-month evaluation of bond failures of orthodontic brackets bonded with direct versus indirect bonding technique: A clinical trial. *Prog. Orthod.* **2014**, *15*, 70. [CrossRef] [PubMed]
11. Swetha, M.; Pai, V.S.; Sanjay, N.; Nandini, S. Indirect versus direct bonding—A shear bond strength comparison: An in vitro study. *J. Contemp. Dent. Pract.* **2011**, *12*, 232–238.
12. McLaughlin, R.P.; Bennett, J.C.; Trevisi, H.J. *Systemized Orthodontic Treatment Mechanics*; Reprinted; Mosby: Edinburgh, UK, 2002; ISBN 0-7234-3171-X.
13. Ciuffolo, F.; Tenisci, N.; Pollutri, L. Modified bonding technique for a standardized and effective indirect bonding procedure. *Am. J. Orthod. Dentofac. Orthop.* **2012**, *141*, 504–509. [CrossRef]
14. Hickham, J.H. Predictable indirect bonding. *J. Clin. Orthod.* **1993**, *27*, 215–217.
15. Gracco, A.; Tracey, S. The insignia system of customized orthodontics. *J. Clin. Orthod.* **2011**, *45*, 442–451. [PubMed]
16. Kalange, J.T. Ideal appliance placement with APC brackets and indirect bonding. *J. Clin. Orthod.* **1999**, *33*, 516–526. [PubMed]
17. Matsuno, I.; Okuda, S.; Nodera, Y. The hybrid core system for indirect bonding. *J. Clin. Orthod.* **2003**, *37*, 160–168.
18. Castilla, A.E.; Crowe, J.J.; Moses, J.R.; Wang, M.; Ferracane, J.L.; Covell, D.A. Measurement and comparison of bracket transfer accuracy of five indirect bonding techniques. *Angle Orthod.* **2014**, *84*, 607–614. [CrossRef]
19. Duarte, M.E.A.; Gribel, B.F.; Spitz, A.; Artese, F.; Miguel, J.A.M. Reproducibility of digital indirect bonding technique using three-dimensional (3D) models and 3D-printed transfer trays. *Angle Orthod.* **2020**, *90*, 92–99. [CrossRef]
20. Niu, Y.; Zeng, Y.; Zhang, Z.; Xu, W.; Xiao, L. Comparison of the transfer accuracy of two digital indirect bonding trays for labial bracket bonding. *Angle Orthod.* **2020**. [CrossRef]
21. Pottier, T.; Brient, A.; Turpin, Y.L.; Chauvel, B.; Meuric, V.; Sorel, O.; Brezulier, D. Accuracy evaluation of bracket repositioning by indirect bonding: Hard acrylic CAD/CAM versus soft one-layer silicone trays, an in vitro study. *Clin. Oral Investig.* **2020**, *24*, 3889–3897. [CrossRef] [PubMed]
22. Zhang, Y.; Yang, C.; Li, Y.; Xia, D.; Shi, T.; Li, C. Comparison of three-dimensional printing guides and double-layer guide plates in accurate bracket placement. *BMC Oral Health* **2020**, *20*, 127. [CrossRef]
23. Koch, P.J. Measuring the accuracy of a computer-aided design and computer-aided manufacturing-based indirect bonding tray. *Am. J. Orthod. Dentofac. Orthop.* **2020**, *158*, 315. [CrossRef] [PubMed]
24. Little, R.M. The Irregularity Index: A quantitative score of mandibular anterior alignment. *Am. J. Orthod.* **1975**, *68*, 554–563. [CrossRef]
25. Koretsi, V.; Kirschbauer, C.; Proff, P.; Kirschneck, C. Reliability and intra-examiner agreement of orthodontic model analysis with a digital caliper on plaster and printed dental models. *Clin. Oral Investig.* **2019**, *23*, 3387–3396. [CrossRef] [PubMed]
26. Becker, K.; Wilmes, B.; Grandjean, C.; Drescher, D. Impact of manual control point selection accuracy on automated surface matching of digital dental models. *Clin. Oral Investig.* **2018**, *22*, 801–810. [CrossRef]
27. R Core Team. *R: A Language and Environment for Statistical Computing*; R Foundation for Statistical Computing: Vienna, Austria, 2018.
28. Cohen, J. *Statistical Power Analysis for the Behavioral Sciences*, 2nd ed.; Taylor and Francis: Hoboken, NJ, USA, 2013; ISBN 9780805802832.
29. Xue, C.; Xu, H.; Guo, Y.; Xu, L.; Dhami, Y.; Wang, H.; Liu, Z.; Ma, J.; Bai, D. Accurate bracket placement using a computer-aided design and computer-aided manufacturing-guided bonding device: An in vivo study. *Am. J. Orthod. Dentofac. Orthop.* **2020**, *157*, 269–277. [CrossRef]
30. Süpple, J.; von Glasenapp, J.; Hofmann, E.; Jost-Brinkmann, P.-G.; Koch, P.J. Accurate bracket placement with an indirect bonding method using digitally designed transfer models printed in different orientations—An in vitro study. *JCM* **2021**, *10*, 2002. [CrossRef] [PubMed]

31. Möhlhenrich, S.C.; Alexandridis, C.; Peters, F.; Kniha, K.; Modabber, A.; Danesh, G.; Fritz, U. Three-dimensional evaluation of bracket placement accuracy and excess bonding adhesive depending on indirect bonding technique and bracket geometry: An in-vitro study. *Head Face Med.* **2020**, *16*, 17. [CrossRef] [PubMed]

32. Grünheid, T.; Lee, M.S.; Larson, B.E. Transfer accuracy of vinyl polysiloxane trays for indirect bonding. *Angle Orthod.* **2016**, *86*, 468–474. [CrossRef]

33. Heo, H.; Kim, M. The effects of orthodontic brackets on the time and accuracy of digital impression taking. *Int. J. Environ. Res. Public Health* **2021**, *18*, 5282. [CrossRef]

34. Kim, Y.-K.; Kim, S.-H.; Choi, T.-H.; Yen, E.H.; Zou, B.; Shin, Y.; Lee, N.-K. Accuracy of intraoral scan images in full arch with orthodontic brackets: A retrospective in vivo study. *Clin. Oral Investig.* **2021**. [CrossRef]

35. Quaas, S.; Loos, R.; Sporbeck, H.; Luthardt, R. Analyse des einflusses der puderapplikation auf die genauigkeit optischer digitalisierungen. *Dtsch. Zahnarztl. Z.* **2005**, *60*, 96–99.

36. Kang, S.-J.; Kee, Y.-J.; Lee, K.C. Effect of the presence of orthodontic brackets on intraoral scans. *Angle Orthod.* **2021**, *91*, 98–104. [CrossRef]

37. Casko, J.S.; Vaden, J.L.; Kokich, V.G.; Damone, J.; James, R.; Cangialosi, T.J.; Riolo, M.L.; Owens, S.E.; Bills, E.D. Objective grading system for dental casts and panoramic radiographs. *Am. J. Orthod. Dentofac. Orthop.* **1998**, *114*, 589–599. [CrossRef]

38. Schmid, J.; Brenner, D.; Recheis, W.; Hofer-Picout, P.; Brenner, M.; Crismani, A.G. Transfer accuracy of two indirect bonding techniques-an in vitro study with 3D scanned models. *Eur. J. Orthod.* **2018**, *40*, 549–555. [CrossRef] [PubMed]

Article

Digital Design of Different Transpalatal Arches Made of Polyether Ether Ketone (PEEK) and Determination of the Force Systems

Cornelia Mieszala [1], Jens Georg Schmidt [2], Kathrin Becker [1,*], Jan Hinrich Willmann [1] and Dieter Drescher [1]

[1] Department of Orthodontics, University of Dusseldorf, 40225 Dusseldorf, Germany; cm@mieszala.de (C.M.); praxis@dr-wilhelmy.de (J.H.W.); d.drescher@uni-duesseldorf.de (D.D.)
[2] Department of Mathematics and Technology, University of Applied Sciences Koblenz, 53424 Remagen, Germany; schmidt@rheinahrcampus.de
[*] Correspondence: kathrin.becker@med.uni-duesseldorf.de; Tel.: +49(0)211-811-8160; Fax: +49(0)211-811-9510

Abstract: The aim of this study was to investigate whether the polymer polyether ether ketone (PEEK), which is approved for (dental) medical appliances, is suitable for the production of orthodontic treatment appliances. Different geometries of transpalatal arches (TPAs) were designed by Computer Aided Design (CAD). Out of a number of different designs and dimensions, four devices were selected and manufactured by milling out of PEEK. A finite element analysis (FEA) and a mechanical in vitro testing were performed to analyze the force systems acting on the first upper molars. Up to an activation (transversal compression) of 4 mm per side (total 8 mm), the PEEK TPAs generated forces between 1.3 and 3.1 Newton (N) in the FEA and between 0.7 and 3.2 N in the mechanical testing. The moments in the oro-vestibular direction were measured between 2.1 and 6.6 Nmm in the FEA and between 1.1 and 6.0 Nmm in the mechanical testing, depending on the individual TPA geometry. With the help of the FEA, it was possible to calculate the von Mises stresses and the deformation patterns of the different TPAs. In some areas, local von Mises stresses exceeded 154–165 MPa, which could lead to a permanent deformation of the respective appliances. In the in vitro testing, however, none of the TPAs showed any visible deformation or fractures. With the help of the FEA and the mechanical testing, it could be shown that PEEK might be suitable as a material for the production of orthodontic TPAs.

Keywords: digital orthodontic appliance; CAD/CAM; polyether ether ketone (PEEK); finite element analysis (FEA); mechanical analysis

Citation: Mieszala, C.; Schmidt, J.G.; Becker, K.; Willmann, J.H.; Drescher, D. Digital Design of Different Transpalatal Arches Made of Polyether Ether Ketone (PEEK) and Determination of the Force Systems . *Appl. Sci.* **2022**, *12* , 1590 . https://doi.org/10.3390/app12031590

Academic Editor: Dorina Lauritano

Received: 22 December 2021
Accepted: 28 January 2022
Published: 2 February 2022

Publisher's Note: MDPI stays neutral with regard to jurisdictional claims in published maps and institutional affiliations.

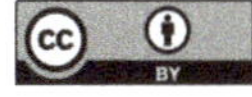

1. Introduction

The transpalatal arch (TPA) is used in orthodontics for three-dimensional adjustment of the molars. The TPA is often used as a passive device to stabilize the molars. However, it can also be employed as an active appliance to expand or compress the dental arch, or to derotate the molars, or to apply differential torque. Usually, the traditional transpalatal arch, according to Goshgarian, is made of 0.9 mm stainless steel wire, which provides a high load-deflection rate [1]. The Goshgarian arch has been modified several times with regard to its material properties and shape. In 1980, Burstone et al. introduced the so-called precision transpalatal arch made of titanium–molybdenum alloy (TMA) [2–4]. The 50% lower Young's modulus of the TMA wire lead to significantly lower force and moments acting on the molars [5] and allowed a wider range of activation [6]. The compound palatal arch developed by Wichelhaus et al. in 2004 was composed of a combination of stainless steel and nickel–titanium elements. The incorporation of the more elastic nickel–titanium elements also reduced the expansion forces and torques [7]. By including superelastic nickel–titanium elements, an expansion up to 4 mm and a derotation of the molars up to 10° could be achieved. Further variants of the classic Goshgarian, as described in the literature [8–10], were designed to create more precise tooth movements and a reduction in the force and moment magnitudes.

Computer Aided Design/ Computer Aided Manufacturing (CAD/CAM) technologies have gained an increasing importance in orthodontics and offer new design and manufacturing possibilities. Whereas metal printing is already established [11–13], only a few studies have investigated the applicability of polyether ether ketone (PEEK) in digital workflows. PEEK is a high-performance polymer with dimensional stability, temperature resistance and excellent biocompatibility [14,15]. The material can be milled and is—with some limitations—also 3D printable [16,17]. Due to its excellent biocompatibility, PEEK was also chosen for dental implants as well as for removable and fixed dentures [18–20]. With its small Young's modulus of 3–5 GPa, PEEK may also be a good candidate for metal-free, aesthetic orthodontic appliances.

Several applications of PEEK in orthodontics have already been reported in the literature. These are mainly passive appliances, such as space maintainers [21] and removable orthodontic retainers [22]. In addition, applications for fixed appliances were proposed [23–26]. However, there is very scarce information as to what extent PEEK is eligible to deliver constant forces and may be used as a replacement for conventional wires or transpalatal arches (TPA) in orthodontics.

Biomechanical properties can be assessed using mechanical testing of 3D-printed specimen, or mathematically by means of finite element analysis (FEA). FEA offers the possibility to simulate and visualize the behavior of complex shapes under mechanical loading. Since FEA can be conducted much faster than mechanical tests, it allows for the assessment of a high number of samples with different shapes. However, since FEA is a numerical approach, it highly depends on material parameters, boundary conditions and the way of modelling. To adjust the underlying parameters and the numerical model, mechanical testing of real samples appears to be mandatory.

The aim of the present study was to investigate whether PEEK is suitable for orthodontic active appliances by assessing the biomechanical properties of a TPA made from PEEK by means of FEA and mechanical testing.

2. Materials and Methods

2.1. Computer-Aided Design (CAD)

A set of digital TPAs with various geometries were designed using the software Blender (version. 2.81) [27]. A randomly selected plaster model was taken from the archive of Department of Orthodontics, University Clinics of Dusseldorf. The plaster model was scanned to gain a digital model. On the first molars, partial shells covering the palatal aspect of the teeth were designed. These shells served to connect the TPAs with the molars. The arches of the TPAs had a horizontal width of 34 mm (from molar to molar), a height of about 14 mm and a distance to the palatal surface of 2 mm on average (Figure 1).

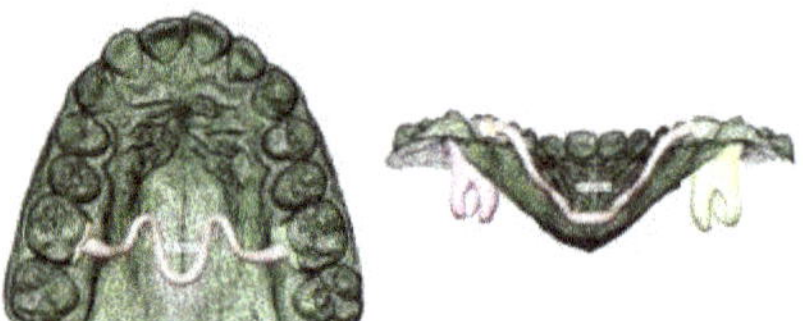

Figure 1. Computer-Aided Design (CAD) of one TPA Geometry.

Out of a number of possible designs, four TPAs were selected that fulfilled common clinical requirements such as patient comfort and mechanical design criteria:

The *Double-arch TPA* consisted of two arches, each having a diameter of 1 mm (Figure 2a). The *Triple-loop-arch TPA* and the *S-bow TPA* were constructed with one connecting element and a diameter of 1.2 mm and 1.5 mm (Figure 2b,c) and the *Omega-loop TPA* showed an oval profile of 1 × 2 mm (Figure 2d). All dimensions are listed in Table 1.

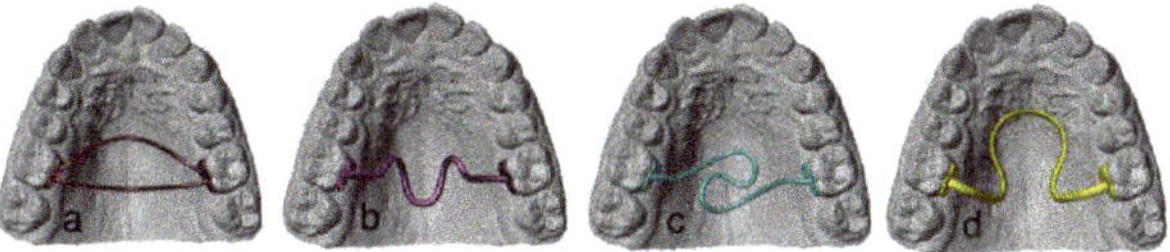

Figure 2. Four different designs of digital TPA Geometries (**a**) Double-arch TPA, (**b**) Triple-loop-arch TPA, (**c**) S-bow TPA, (**d**) Omega-loop TPA.

Table 1. Dimensions of the four different designs: horizontal (x-axis), sagittal (y-axis), vertical (z-axis), arch diameter and number of the elements in the FEA.

Dimensions (mm)	Double-Arch TPA	Triple-Loop-Arch TPA	S-Bow TPA	Omega-Loop TPA
Horizontal	34	34	34	34
Sagittal	13	11	14	20
Vertical	14	14	14.5	10
Cross section	1 each	1.5	1.2	1×2
Number of elements in the FEA	155,578	136,341	167,257	151,933

2.2. Creating of High-Quality Meshes

For the FEA, the meshes of the digital TPAs (Figure 3a), were triangulated and converted into meshes with high element quality using the Meshmixer program (version 3.4.35, 2017, Autodesk Meshmixer RRID:SCR_015736) (Figure 3b) and the MeshLab software (version 2016.12, https://www.meshlab.net, last accessed on 1 November 2021) for mesh corrections and optimizations (Figure 3c).

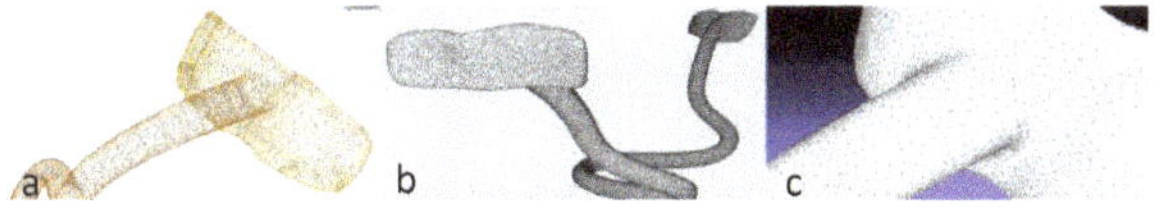

Figure 3. Mesh creation and optimization (**a**) Blender, (**b**) Meshmixer, (**c**) MeshLab.

2.3. Finite Element Analysis (FEA)

The FEA was performed using the software FEBio (developed by SA Maas, BJ Ellis, GA Ateshian, JA Weiss) [28]. The pre-processor (FEBio-PreView, version 2.13) was used to build the finite element model and to define the boundary conditions. In order to guarantee an acceptable mesh quality, we bounded—for every tetrahedron—the ratio of the diameter of the circumsphere R and the length of the shortest edge L by the ratio $R/L < 1.4$. The number of the elements for each appliance are listed in Table 1.

The FE solver (FEBio-Run) was used to perform the calculations, and the post-processor (FEBio-PostView, version 2.4.4) was employed for visualization.

For the present study, the material parameters of the PEEK material were set to a Young's modulus of 5.1 GPa and a Poisson's ratio of 0.42, according to the parameters provided by the manufacturer of the material used for fabrication [29].

As boundary conditions, an activation in the horizontal plane between the two molar shells from 1 mm up to an expansion of 8 mm (4 mm per site) was defined, and computed in steps of 1 mm displacement each. The forces and moments acting at the point of force application (PF) on the inner surfaces of the shells (at the first upper molars), were determined. In addition, resulting moments at the centers of resistance (CR) were assessed. Moments around the vertical axis were considered to be *rotatory*, around the oro-vestibular axis to be *angulatory* and around the mesio-distal axis to account for *tipping* movements.

2.4. Computer-Aided Manufacturing (CAM)

The manufacturing of the four different PEEK TPAs were carried out by the dental laboratory "Dentes" (Dentes Fräszentrum GmbH, Neuss, Germany). The files were prepared for milling with the dental CAM system ZYKLONcam (KON-AN- TEC, Münster, Germany) and milled out of a PEEK disc from Merz Dental (PEEK BioSolution white, Merz Dental GmbH, Lütjeburg, Germany) with a 5-axis milling machine CORiTEC 350i Loader (Imes-icore GmbH, Eiterfeld, Germany). The support structures, which were necessary for fixation of the TPAs while milling, were carefully removed. No further finishing was required.

2.5. Set-Up of the Mechanical Testing

The mechanical in vitro test was performed by measurement system RMSBiomech, which consisted of a robotic arm, a force-moment sensor and an adjustable table (Figure 4a). Each of the TPAs was glued (Pattex, epoxy resin 2-component adhesive, Henkel, Germany) to custom designed and 3D printed fixation device (Figure 4b) made of a polyamide, printed by PROTIQ (Blomberg, Germany) and representing the original molars. The fixation devices were screwed to the sensor to allow measurement of the 3D forces and moments. The setup was constructed such that only the upper right first molar was movable, whereas the contralateral molar stayed attached to the table.

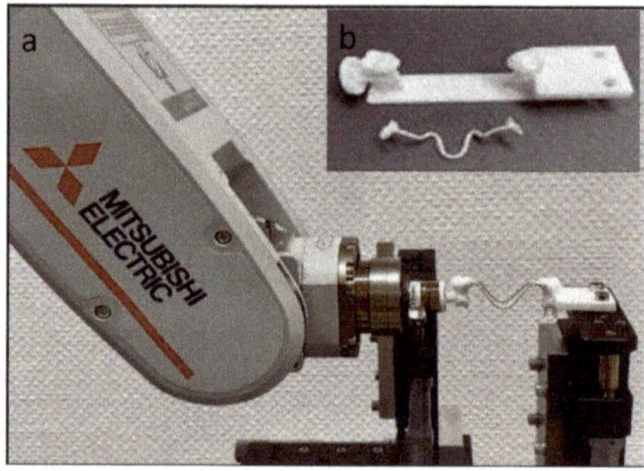

Figure 4. Experimental setup of the mechanical in vitro testing; (**a**) Robotic arm with supersensitive force–moment sensor and position table; (**b**) 3D printed polyamide fixation device with one TPA, milled out of PEEK.

The measurement of the forces and the moments was carried out by a 6-axis force-moment sensor (FT Nano17, Schunk, Lauffen/Neckar, Germany), which was connected to the robotic arm via a magnetic attachment. The computer controlled robotic arm (Mitsubishi Electric, MELFA, RV-2FR, Ratingen, Germany) was capable of movements using all six spatial degrees of freedom.

2.6. Mechanical Testing

The software RMSBiomech controlling the robot stored the activation distance as well as the measured force Fx, Fy, Fz and moment components Mx, My, Mz. Each TPA was activated identical to the previous FEA in compression mode (8 mm in total, 4 mm per side) perpendicular to the mid-sagittal plane. Forces and moments were recorded in 0.1 mm steps from 1 to 8 mm of activation. This procedure was repeated ten times to calculate the mean values. The measured forces and moments represented those acting at the inner surfaces of the shells (PF) or the molars, respectively. The moments acting on the center of resistance (CR) were computed, assuming the CR to be positioned at 7 mm apically to the point of force application (PF), i.e., approximately 1–2 mm below the tri-furcation of the upper right molar [30,31].

3. Results

The results of the Finite Element Analysis and the mechanical testing were measured in all three dimensions and are reported in Table 2.

Table 2. a–d Measurements of the finite element analysis and the mechanical testing; Forces: Fx (transversal), Fy (sagittal), Fz (vertical); Moments: Mx (angulation), My (buccal tipping), Mz (rotation); von Mises stresses; (a) Double-arch TPA, (b) Triple-loop-arch TPA, (c) S-bow TPA, (d) Omega-loop TPA.

| | Finite Element Analysis | | | | | | | | | | Mechanical Testing | | | | | |
| Activation (mm) | Forces | | | Moments at the Point of Force Application (PF) | | | Moments at the Center of Resistance (CR) | | | von Mises Stress [MPa] | Forces | | | Moments at the Center of Resistance (CR) | | |
	Fx (N) FEA	Fy(N) FEA	Fz (N) FEA	Mx Nmm FEA.	My Nmm FEA	Mz Nmm FEA	Mx Nmm FEA	My Nmm FEA	Mz Nmm FEA		Fx (N) test	Fy(N) test	Fz (N) test	Mx Nmm test	My Nmm test	Mz Nmm test
								(a) Double-arch TPA								
0.5	0.5	0	0	0	−3	−0.5	0	0.9	0.3		0.4	0	0	−0.1	0.5	0.1
1	0.9	0	0	−0.1	−7	−1.3	0	1.6	0.5	46	0.7	0	0.1	−0.1	0.8	0.2
1.5	1.3	0	0	−0.2	−10	−2	0	2	0.7		1.1	0	0.1	−0.1	1.1	0.4
2	1.7	0	0.1	−0.2	−13	−2.5	0	2.3	0.8	89	1.4	0	0.1	−0.1	1.3	0.5
2.5	2.1	0	0.1	−0.3	−16	−3	−0.1	2.4	0.9		1.6	0	0.1	−0.1	1.3	0.7
3	2.5	0.1	0.1	−0.3	−20	−3.8	−0.1	2.4	1.0	128	1.9	0	0.2	−0.1	1.3	0.9
3.5	2.8	0.1	0.1	−0.4	−23	−4.5	−0.1	2.3	1.0		2.1	0	0.2	−0.1	1.2	1.1
4	3.2	0.1	0.1	−0.5	−26	−5	−0.1	2.1	1.0	165	2.3	0.1	0.2	−0.2	1.1	1.3
								(b) Triple-loop-arch TPA								
0.5	0.4	0	0	−0.1	−4	0.1	0	−0.5	0.8		0.5	0	0	0	−0.5	−0.7
1	0.7	0	0	−0.1	−8	0.2	−0.1	−1.1	1.7	43	1.0	0	0	0	−1.1	−1.3
1.5	1.1	0	0.1	−0.2	−11	0.3	−0.1	−1.8	2.4		1.4	0	0.1	0	−1.7	−1.9
2	1.4	0	0.1	−0.2	−15	0.5	−0.2	−2.7	3.2	83	1.8	0	0.1	0.1	−2.5	−2.5
2.5	1.7	0	0.1	−0.3	−18	0.5	−0.2	−3.5	3.9		2.2	0	0.1	0.1	−3.3	−3.1
3	2.0	0	0.1	−0.3	−21	0.7	−0.3	−4.5	4.6	120	2.6	0	0.1	0.2	−4.2	−3.7
3.5	2.3	0	0.1	−0.4	−25	0.9	−0.4	−5.5	5.3		2.9	0	0.1	0.2	−5.1	−4.2
4	2.5	0	0.1	−0.4	−29	1	−0.4	−6.5	6.0	154	3.2	0	0.1	0.2	−6.0	−4.7
								(c) S-bow TPA								
0.5	0.3	0	0	−0.1	−3	0.2	0	−0.4	0.7		0.2	0	0	0.0	−0.2	−0.3
1	0.5	0	0	−0.1	−5.5	0.3	0	−1.0	1.3	42	0.3	0	0	0.0	−0.5	−0.6
1.5	0.8	0	0	−0.1	−8	0.4	0	−1.7	1.8		0.5	0	0	0.0	−0.8	−0.8
2	1.0	0	0	−0.2	−11	0.5	0	−2.5	2.3	81	0.6	0	0	−0.1	−1.1	−1.1
2.5	1.2	0	0	−0.2	−14	0.5	0.1	−3.4	2.8		0.8	0	0	−0.1	−1.6	−1.3
3	1.4	0.1	0.1	−0.2	−17	0.5	0.2	−4.4	3.2	119	0.9	0	0	−0.2	−2.1	−1.4
3.5	1.6	0.1	0.1	−0.3	−19	0.5	0.2	−5.5	3.5		1.0	0	0	−0.3	−2.6	−1.5
4	1.7	0.1	0.1	−0.3	−22	0.5	0.3	−6.6	3.7	154	1.1	0	0	−0.3	−3.2	−1.7

Table 2. *Cont.*

Activation (mm)	Finite Element Analysis									von Mises Stress [MPa]	Mechanical Testing					
	Forces			Moments at the Point of Force Application (PF)			Moments at the Center of Resistance (CR)				Forces			Moments at the Center of Resistance (CR)		
	Fx (N) FEA	Fy(N) FEA	Fz (N) FEA	Mx Nmm FEA.	My Nmm FEA	Mz Nmm FEA	Mx Nmm FEA	My Nmm FEA	Mz Nmm FEA		Fx (N) test	Fy(N) test	Fz (N) test	Mx Nmm test	My Nmm test	Mz Nmm test
										(d) Omega-loop TPA						
0.5	**0.2**	**0**	**0**	0	−1	−0.7	0	0.4	−0.4		**0.1**	**0**	**0**	0.0	0.1	0.3
1	**0.3**	**0**	**0**	0	−2	−1.4	0	0.8	−0.7	17	**0.2**	**0**	**0**	0.0	0.3	0.6
1.5	**0.5**	**0**	**0**	0	−3	−2	0	1.2	−1.1		**0.3**	**0**	**0**	0.0	0.5	0.9
2	**0.7**	**0**	**0**	0	−4	−2.7	0	1.5	−1.5	35	**0.4**	**0**	**0**	0.0	0.6	1.1
2.5	**0.8**	**0**	**0**	0	−5	−3.4	0	1.8	−1.8		**0.5**	**0**	**0**	0.1	0.8	1.4
3	**1.0**	**0**	**0**	−0.1	−7	−4	0	2.0	−2.2	51	**0.6**	**0**	**0**	0.1	0.9	1.7
3.5	**1.1**	**0**	**0**	−0.1	−8	−4.7	0.1	2.2	−2.6		**0.6**	**0**	**0**	0.1	1.0	2.0
4	**1.3**	**0**	**0**	−0.1	−9	−5.4	0.1	2.4	−2.9	68	**0.7**	**0**	**0**	0.1	1.1	2.3

3.1. Finite Element Analysis

At a maximum activation of 4 mm per side in the transversal axis, the *Double-arch TPA* with two arches of 1 mm diameter each, generated the highest forces (3.1 Newton (N) per side). The *Triple-loop-arch TPA* and the *S-bow TPA*, both with a round diameter of 1.2 mm and 1.5 mm, generated 2.5 and 1.7 N per side. The *Omega-loop TPA* with an oval diameter of 1 × 2 mm and a big loop generated 1.3 N per side, the lowest force. In the sagittal and vertical direction, negligible forces less than 0.01 N were found.

The applied and resulting moments were assessed at CR and PF at the inner surface of the shell, palatal to the dental crown of the upper right molar. Overall, the highest moments were found around the mesio-distal axis representing a buccal *tipping*.

At the maximum activation of 4 mm per side, at CR, moments ranged from 2.1 Nmm (*Double-arch TPA*) to −6.6 Nmm (*S-bow TPA*), and, at PF, the moments ranged from −9 Nmm (*Omega-loop TPA*) to −29 Nmm (*Triple-loop-arch TPA*). The *rotatory* moments around the vertical axis reached a maximum of 6 Nmm (*Triple-loop-arch TPA)* at CR and −5.4 Nmm (*Omega-loop TPA*) at PF. The *angulation*, i.e., moments around the oro-vestibular axis, were very small for all treatment appliance with absolute values less than 0.5 Nmm. Figure 5a, b summarizes the *buccal tipping* at PF and CR for the investigated TPAs.

The FEA enabled calculation of the von Mises stresses for each TPA variant. Up to an activation of 3 mm per side, the local von Mises stresses ranged from 51 to 128 MPa and sometimes slightly exceeded the yield point from PEEK of 120 MPa. Upon further activation of the TPAs up to 4 mm, three appliances produced local von Mises stress clearly above the yield point (*S-bow TPA* and *Triple-loop-arch TPA*: 154 MPa and *Double-arch TPA*: 165 MPa). The von Mises stresses for the different TPA variants are visualized in Figure 6 for a bilateral activation of 4 mm. It can be seen that the highest material stresses occurred at the interface between the TPA and the shells (marked in red-orange).

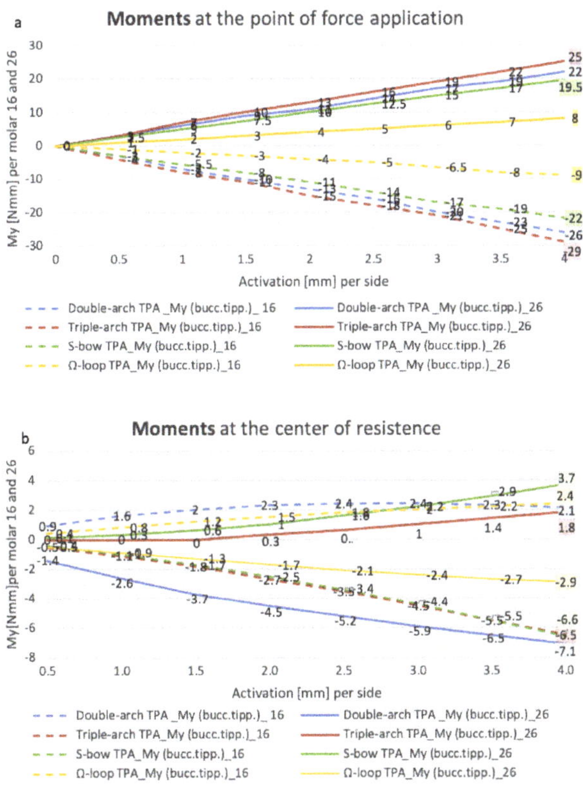

Figure 5. (a,b) FEA, resulting moments in Newton millimeter (Nmm) for buccal tipping per molar 16 (dashed line) and 26 (continuous line) measured by transversal activation of 0.5 to 4 mm per side; (**a**) at the point of force application; (**b**) at the center of resistance.

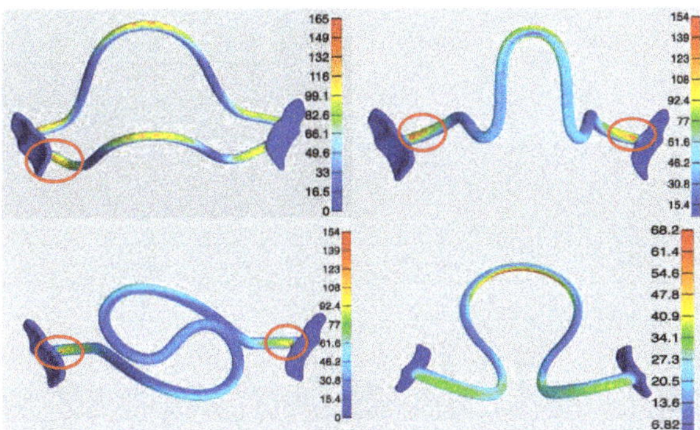

Figure 6. FEA, graphical illustration of the von Mises stress at a maximum of 4 mm bilateral activation per side. The side scale indicates the corresponding numerical data (here: megapascals) to the color gradient, blue shows the lowest stress and red the highest stress (areas marked in red-orange).

The displacement in the sagittal direction differed depending on the TPA geometry: Anterior movement was seen for the *Double-arch TPA* and the *Omega-loop TPA* (1.3 mm and 0.5 mm), whereas distal displacement was seen for the *Triple-loop-arch TPA* (−0.5 mm). A different pattern was seen for the *S-bow TPA* where one side moved to the anterior, and the other in a distal direction (1.5 mm and −2 mm). In the apical direction, movements ranged from −1.5 mm (*Omega-loop TPA*) to −3.9 mm (*S-bow TPA*).

Figure 7 summarizes the deformation pattern of the four TPAs in all three dimensions. It can be seen that apical displacement was most pronounced for the *S-bow TPA* and the *Double-arch TPA*, reaching 3.9 mm and 2.7 mm, respectively.

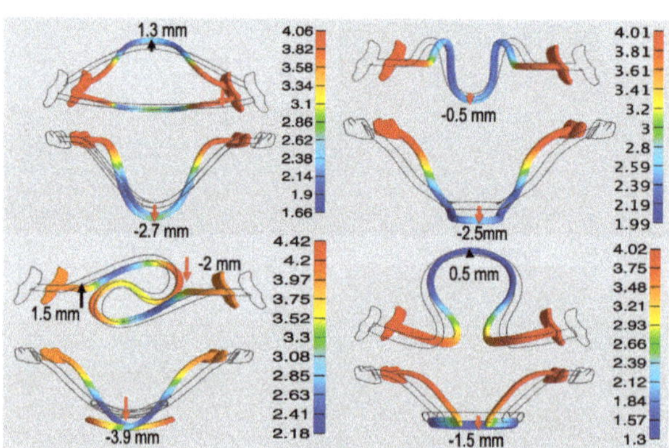

Figure 7. FEA, graphical visualization of the deformation pattern at a maximum of 4 mm bilateral activation per side. The side scale indicates the corresponding numerical values (here: millimeters) to the color gradient, blue indicates the smallest movement and red the largest.

3.2. Mechanical Testing

The resulting forces and moments of the mechanical testing were measured in all three dimensions and are shown in Table 2. In contrast to the FEA, the *Triple-loop-arch TPA* showed the highest forces (3.2 N per side) and the *Double-arch TPA* the second highest forces (2,3 N per side) at an activation of 4 mm per side. Likewise, to the FEA, the *S-bow TPA* and the *Omega-loop TPA* generated lower forces per side (1.1 N per side and 0.7 N). Figure 8 compares the resulting forces from the FEA with the mechanical tests of the investigated TPAs. In the sagittal and apical direction, negligible forces smaller than 0.2 N were identified.

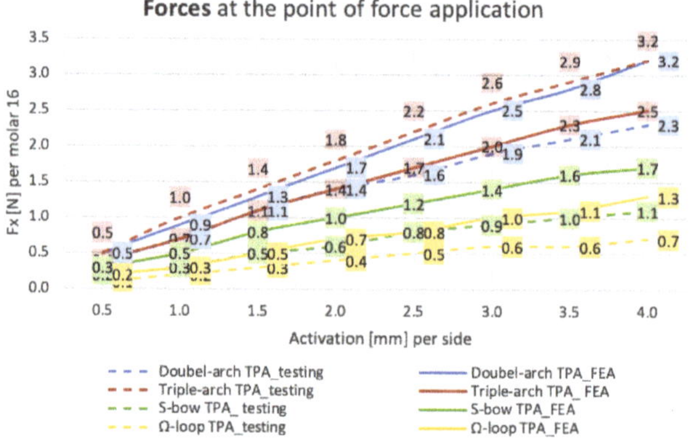

Figure 8. Mechanical test (dashed line) vs. FEA (continuous line): resulting forces in Newton (N) in oro-vestibular direction per molar by transversal activation of 0.5 to 4 mm per side.

For the mechanical testing, resulting moments were assessed only at the CR. Similar to the FEA, the highest moments occurred around the mesio-distal axis representing a *buccal tipping* ranging from 1.1 Nmm (*Double-arch TPA*) to −6 Nmm (*Triple-loop-arch TPA*). The *rotatory* moments around the vertical axis ranged from 1.3 Nmm (*Double-arch TPA*) to −4.7 Nmm (*Triple-loop-arch TPA*). The *angulation*, around the oro-vestibular axis, was lowest and ranged from 0.1 to −0.3 Nmm for all appliances.

4. Discussion

Digital workflows and computer-aided design (CAD) are transforming the daily work in all dental disciplines. In orthodontics, they enable the provision of individualized appliances designed specifically to the patient's needs.

Owing to the advancement of computer-aided manufacturing (CAM), new materials for 3D printing or 5-axis milling are becoming available [32]. Most of the printable polymers currently available on the dental market are limited to temporary use in the mouth. In orthodontics, they are utilized for insertion guides of orthodontic mini-implants [33,34] or surgical splints for orthognathic surgery [35]. Fully digitally planned and CAM-fabricated appliances made of printed or milled materials have been described in the literature. They are utilized for active treatment and retention purposes [11–13,36–38].

The biocompatible high-performance polymer polyether ether ketone (PEEK) that was analyzed in the present study has been used in dentistry for dental implants [18–20] as well as for permanent and removable dentures [14,15]. In the orthodontic field, PEEK has been tested for the manufacturing of removable and fixed space maintainers. Owing to the low modulus of elasticity, it has also been tested for orthodontic wires made of or covered by PEEK [23–25]. Therefore, the present study investigated whether PEEK could also be suitable for the CAM fabrication of transpalatal arches.

In contrast to the traditional transpalatal arch made of stainless steel or TMA wire, the use of digital design programs enables the user to create customized and precise treatment appliances for specific needs. The TPA geometries presented in this article reflect the wide range of design possibilities.

PEEK, in contrast to stainless steel (160 GPa) or TMA (80 GPa), has a significantly lower Young's modulus of only 3 to 5 GPa. When employed as a material for orthodontic purposes, forces and moments of much smaller magnitudes can be expected. Accordingly, the activation range of the TPAs made out of PEEK that were measured in the present study was considerably higher compared to values previously reported for TPAs made of stainless steel (maximum activation < 3 mm) or TMA (maximum activation < 5–6 mm).

Up to an activation of 6 mm, none of the TPA geometries presented in this study exceeded the recommended force limit of 2.5 N [5]. The *S-bow TPA* and the *Omega-loop TPA* generated expansion forces below 1.5 N up to an activation of 8 mm, implicating that a further activation would be conceivable for the respective geometries.

Out of the TPAs tested in this study, the *Double-arch TPA* and the *Triple-loop-arch TPA* generated the highest forces, which were in the range of 2.5 to 3.0 N and appeared appropriate for orthodontic purposes. Among the two, the *Double-arch TPA* showed rather low moments and could thus be well suited for expansion or—possibly with an enlarged or modified cross section—also as an anchorage unit. The *Triple-loop-arch TPA* generated similar forces but higher moments (rotation −6.6 Nmm) and may therefore also be suited for molar derotation. The *S-bow TPA* generated lower forces and higher moments (rotation 3 to 6 Nmm), which may in principle be eligible for orthodontic treatment. However, the FEA revealed that the two "S" arches might end up in direct contact upon higher activation, which has to be considered in the case of clinical application. The *Omega-loop-arch TPA*, with its large spring, generated very low forces (about 1.0 N) and may therefore not be useful for expansion or for anchorage.

The traditional TPA made of stainless steel or TMA is usually connected to the molars via palatal attachments. This plug-in connection has the advantage that the palatal arch can be easily removed and re-inserted for activation. However, a limitation of this approach is related to the slot play leading to undesirable side effects, such as the unwanted reduction in torque moments [5,7] Another limitation of conventional TPAs is related to the fact that their frequent re-activation is required.

The CAD/CAM-fabricated TPAs consist of one piece and should be directly bonded to the palatal surface of the molars. Due to the high dimensional stability of the palatal connection from the arch to the tooth, side effects can be reduced and three-dimensional tooth movements can be achieved in a more precise manner. Due to the large activation range, regularly re-activating of the TPAs might not be necessary.

Comparable to the activation of TPAs made of stainless steel [8], three out of four TPAs made of PEEK exceeded the yield point at a bilateral activation of 4 mm in the FEA, whereas this did not occur for a bilateral activation of 3 mm. Accordingly, we can expect that higher activations may lead to an irreversible deformation during insertion. In this case, the TPAs made out of PEEK might not recover completely. Consequently, the intended tooth movement might not be carried out to the full extent. In the mechanical in vitro analysis, however, none of the PEEK TPAs investigated in this study showed any visible deformation. Hence, for the geometries investigated, the maximum activation ranges of the PEEK TPAs are most likely to be in a range slightly below 4 mm per side.

On average, the values measured in the mechanical in vitro testing for the force systems were lower than the values calculated in the FEA. Only one appliance (*Triple-loop-arch TPA*) showed higher values in the test than in the FEA. Possibly, this could be related to the fact that a linear elasticity of the PEEK material was assumed for the FEA. However, the PEEK material—as with most polymers—shows a non-linear behavior above a certain load. Therefore, a change in the material structure of the PEEK polymer during activation (horizontal compression) and an incomplete recovery of the material in the mechanical testing may occur. It may be speculated that this could be the reason for the lower forces in the in vitro testing, and future studies are required to further investigate this aspect.

The FEA revealed that the highest material stresses occurred at the junction of the connecting elements to the shells. Using CAD-supported planning at this point, the user has the possibility to strengthen the TPAs in the areas with the highest material stress. This might lead to a reduction in the material stress when subjected to similar force systems.

Finally, with the help of the FEA, it was possible to obtain information on the deformation of each treatment appliance in all three dimensions. It was observed that greater transversal activation leads to significant apical movement of the treatment appliance from 1.5 up to almost 4 mm, depending on the TPA geometry. A palatal distance of about 2 mm, as described in this study, of the TPAs would result in contact with the palatal mucosa during insertion. This fact should be kept in mind in the virtual planning of the TPAs designed by CAD.

5. Conclusions

The present study showed that CAD–CAM-manufactured transpalatal arches (TPA) made of PEEK might be a promising alternative to conventional materials.

The FEA was found to be suitable to investigate the mechanical behavior of different CAD/CAM-fabricated TPA geometries. The mechanical in vitro analysis supplemented the FEA by enabling measurement of the forces and moments acting on both molars simultaneously. In combination with the FEA, predictions about the force systems acting on the molars by CAD/CAM-fabricated PEEK TPAs could be obtained in all three dimensions.

The TPA geometries presented in this study showed clinically appropriate expansion forces up to 3 N per side. Due to the low load-deflection rate of the flexible PEEK material, the activation ranges are much higher in comparison to conventional TPAs. The four different geometries utilized in the study reflect the wide variability in design options. The *Triple-loop-arch TPA* with a force system ranging from 2.5 to about 3 N appeared to be most appropriate for the application of moments, whereas the *Double-arch TPA*, which delivered force systems of comparable magnitude, seemed to be most appropriate for the expansion as well as anchorage of the molars. In the future, the development of customized TPAs for specific patients' needs might become possible using CAD.

The practical benefits of CAD/CAM-fabricated appliances are currently advancing owing to the development of novel 3D-printable materials and improvements in CAD software. However, their introduction to clinical settings requires validation of their eligibility by means of simulated and biomechanical testing, and analysis of biocompatibility. Whereas PEEK has already demonstrated its suitability for permanent use in the mouth, only a few studies have assessed its applicability as a retention device in orthodontics. This study presented that PEEK may also be effective as a CAD–CAM-fabricated active orthodontic appliance and might offer a metal-free, aesthetic alternative to conventional approaches. As the 5-axis milling out of a PEEK disc is associated with a high material loss, improvements in additive 3D printing technology will most likely reduce costs in the future.

The behavior of PEEK under in vivo (intraoral) conditions should be evaluated in future experimental studies.

Author Contributions: C.M.: Conceptualization, methodology, formal analysis, investigation, writing—original draft preparation. D.D.: Conceptualization, methodology, formal analysis, investigation, writing—review and editing. J.G.S.: methodology, software, visualization, formal analysis. J.H.W.: Conceptualization, methodology, project administration. K.B.: Conceptualization, writing—original draft preparation, writing—review and editing. All authors have read and agreed to the published version of the manuscript.

Funding: This research received no external funding.

Institutional Review Board Statement: The present study was approved by the ethical committee of the University of Dusseldorf (Ref. no. 2019-643, date of approval: 4 September 2019).

Informed Consent Statement: Not applicable.

Data Availability Statement: Data will be provided upon reasonable request.

Acknowledgments: The authors thank the dental laboratory "Dentes" (Fräszentrum GmbH, Neuss, Germany) for their kind support in the manufacturing of the different TPAs.

Conflicts of Interest: The authors declare no conflict of interest.

References

1. Baldini, G.; Luder, H.U. Influence of Arch Shape on the Transverse Effects of Transpalatal Arches of the Goshgarian Type during Application of Buccal Root Torque. *Am. J. Orthod.* **1982**, *81*, 202–208. [CrossRef]
2. Burstone, C.J.; Koenig, H.A. Precision Adjustment of the Transpalatal Lingual Arch: Computer Arch Form Predetermination. *Am. J. Orthod.* **1981**, *79*, 115–133. [CrossRef]
3. Burstone, C.J.; Manhartsberger, C. Precision Lingual Arches. Passive Applications. *Am. J. Orthod.* **1981**, *80*, 1–16. [CrossRef]
4. Burstone, C.J. Precision Lingual Arches. Active Applications. *J. Clin. Orthod. JCO* **1989**, *23*, 101–109.
5. Hoederath, H.; Bourauel, C.; Drescher, D. Differences between Two Transpalatal Arch Systems upon First-, Second-, and Third-Order Bending Activation. *J. Orofac. Orthop. Fortschr. Kieferorthopädie* **2001**, *62*, 58–73. [CrossRef]
6. Tsetsilas, M.; Konermann, A.-C.; Keilig, L.; Reimann, S.; Jäger, A.; Bourauel, C. Symmetric and Asymmetric Expansion of Molars Using a Burstone-Type Transpalatal Arch. *J. Orofac. Orthop. Fortschritte Kieferorthopädie* **2015**, *76*, 377–390. [CrossRef]
7. Wichelhaus, A.; Sander, C.; Sander, F.G. Development and Biomechanical Investigation of a New Compound Palatal Arch. *J. Orofac. Orthop. Kieferorthopädie* **2004**, *65*, 104–122. [CrossRef]
8. Gündüz, E.; Crismani, A.G.; Bantleon, H.P.; Hönigl, K.D.; Zachrisson, B.U. An Improved Transpalatal Bar Design. Part II. Clinical Upper Molar Derotation—Case Report. *Angle Orthod.* **2003**, *73*, 244–248. [CrossRef]
9. Ambrositsch, P.; Bantleon, H.-P. Der S-Garian TPA—Einsatzmöglichkeiten und Vorteile des Transpalatinalbogendesigns. *Informationen Aus Orthod. Kieferorthopädie* **2016**, *48*, 7–10. [CrossRef]
10. Nikkerdar, A. Butterfly Arch: A Device for Precise Controlling of the Upper Molars in Three Planes of Space. *J. Dent. Tehran Iran.* **2013**, *10*, 221–226.
11. Graf, S.; Vasudavan, S.; Wilmes, B. CAD/CAM Metallic Printing of a Skeletally Anchored Upper Molar Distalizer. *J. Clin. Orthod. JCO* **2020**, *54*, 140–150.
12. Graf, S.; Cornelis, M.A.; Hauber Gameiro, G.; Cattaneo, P.M. Computer-Aided Design and Manufacture of Hyrax Devices: Can We Really Go Digital? *Am. J. Orthod. Dentofac. Orthop.* **2017**, *152*, 870–874. [CrossRef]
13. Graf, S.; Vasudavan, S.; Wilmes, B. CAD-CAM Design and 3-Dimensional Printing of Mini-Implant Retained Orthodontic Appliances. *Am. J. Orthod. Dentofac. Orthop.* **2018**, *154*, 877–882. [CrossRef]

14. Skirbutis, G. PEEK Polymer's Properties and Its Use in Prosthodontics. A Review. *Stomatol. Balt. Dent. Maxillofac. J.* **2018**, *20*, 54–58.

15. Alexakou, E. PEEK High Performance Polymers: A Review of Properties and Clinical Applications in Prosthodontics and Restorative Dentistry. *Eur. J. Prosthodont. Restor. Dent.* **2019**, *27*, 113–121. [CrossRef]

16. Jockusch, J.; Özcan, M. Additive Manufacturing of Dental Polymers: An Overview on Processes, Materials and Applications. *Dent. Mater. J.* **2020**, *39*, 345–354. [CrossRef]

17. Wang, Y.; Müller, W.-D.; Rumjahn, A.; Schwitalla, A. Parameters Influencing the Outcome of Additive Manufacturing of Tiny Medical Devices Based on PEEK. *Mater. Basel Switz.* **2020**, *13*, 466. [CrossRef]

18. Schwitalla, A.; Müller, W.-D. PEEK Dental Implants: A Review of the Literature. *J. Oral Implantol.* **2013**, *39*, 743–749. [CrossRef]

19. Whitty, T. PEEK—A New Material for CAD/CAM Dentistry. *eLABORATE* **2014**, 32–36. Available online: https://panadent.co.uk/wp-content/uploads/2014/11/PEEK-A-new-material-for-CADCAM-dentistry.pdf (accessed on 21 November 2021).

20. Mendes, J.M.; Botelho, P.C.; Mendes, J.; Barreiros, P.; Aroso, C.; Silva, A.S. Comparison of Fracture Strengths of Three Provisional Prosthodontic CAD/CAM Materials: Laboratory Fatigue Tests. *Appl. Sci.* **2021**, *11*, 9589. [CrossRef]

21. Ierardo, G.; Luzzi, V.; Lesti, M.; Vozza, I.; Brugnoletti, O.; Polimeni, A.; Bossu, M. Peek Polymer in Orthodontics: A Pilot Study on Children. *J. Clin. Exp. Dent.* **2017**, *9*, e1271–e1275. [CrossRef]

22. Xepapadeas, A.B.; Weise, C.; Frank, K.; Spintzyk, S.; Poets, C.F.; Wiechers, C.; Arand, J.; Koos, B. Technical Note on Introducing a Digital Workflow for Newborns with Craniofacial Anomalies Based on Intraoral Scans—Part I: 3D Printed and Milled Palatal Stimulation Plate for Trisomy 21. *BMC Oral Health* **2020**, *20*, 20. [CrossRef] [PubMed]

23. Shirakawa, N.; Iwata, T.; Miyake, S.; Otuka, T.; Koizumi, S.; Kawata, T. Mechanical Properties of Orthodontic Wires Covered with a Polyether Ether Ketone Tube. *Angle Orthod.* **2018**, *88*, 442–449. [CrossRef] [PubMed]

24. Tada, Y.; Hayakawa, T.; Nakamura, Y. Load-Deflection and Friction Properties of PEEK Wires as Alternative Orthodontic Wires. *Materials* **2017**, *10*, 914. [CrossRef] [PubMed]

25. Maekawa, M.; Kanno, Z.; Wada, T.; Hongo, T.; Doi, H.; Hanawa, T.; Ono, T.; Uo, M. Mechanical Properties of Orthodontic Wires Made of Super Engineering Plastic. *Dent. Mater. J.* **2015**, *34*, 114–119. [CrossRef]

26. Krey, K.-F. 3D-Printed Orthodontic Brackets—Proof of Concept Dreidimensional Gedruckte Kieferorthopädische Brackets—Eine Machbarkeitsstudie. *Int. J. Comput. Dent.* **2016**, *19*, 351–362. [PubMed]

27. Community, B.O. *Blender—A 3D Modelling and Rendering Package*; Stichting Blender Foundation: Amsterdam, The Netherlands, 2018; Available online: http://www.blender.org (accessed on 30 July 2020).

28. Maas, S.A.; Ellis, B.J.; Ateshian, G.A.; Weiss, J.A. FEBio: Finite elements for biomechanics. *J. Biomech. Eng.* **2012**, *134*, 011005. [CrossRef]

29. Available online: https://www.merz-dental.de/fileadmin/user_upload/downloads/IFU/GBA_PEEK_BioSolution_907187-2021-08-05_907260-2021-10-02_907328-2021-09-01.pdf (accessed on 10 September 2019).

30. Schwindling, F.-P. Vom Centroid zur Widerstandszone. *Kieferorthopädie* **2020**, *34*, 39–46.

31. Viecilli, R.F.; Budiman, A.; Burstone, C.J. Axes of Resistance for Tooth Movement: Does the Center of Resistance Exist in 3-Dimensional Space? *Am. J. Orthod. Dentofac. Orthop.* **2013**, *143*, 163–172. [CrossRef]

32. Scribante, A.; Gallo, S.; Pascadopoli, M.; Canzi, P.; Marconi, S.; Montasser, M.A.; Bressani, D.; Gandini, P.; Sfondrini, M.F. Properties of CAD/CAM 3D Printing Dental Materials and Their Clinical Applications in Orthodontics: Where Are We Now? *Appl. Sci.* **2022**, *12*, 551. [CrossRef]

33. Wilmes, B.; Vasudavan, S.; Drescher, D. CAD-CAM–Fabricated Mini-Implant Insertion Guides for the Delivery of a Distalization Appliance in a Single Appointment. *Am. J. Orthod. Dentofac. Orthop.* **2019**, *156*, 148–156. [CrossRef] [PubMed]

34. Gabriele, O.D.; Dallatana, G.; Riva, R.; Vasudavan, S.; Wilmes, B. The Easy Driver for Placement of Palatal Mini-Implants and a Maxillary Expander in a Single Appointment. *J. Clin. Orthod.* **2017**, *51*, 728–737. [PubMed]

35. Brauer, L.; Pausch, N. Digital unterstützte kombiniert kieferorthopädisch-kieferchirurgische Therapie. *Zahnmed. Up2date* **2018**, *12*, 215–234. [CrossRef]

36. Al Mortadi, N.; Eggbeer, D.; Lewis, J.; Williams, R.J. CAD/CAM/AM Applications in the Manufacture of Dental Appliances. *Am. J. Orthod. Dentofacial Orthop.* **2012**, *142*, 727–733. [CrossRef]

37. Wolf, M.; Schumacher, P.; Jäger, F.; Wego, J.; Fritz, U.; Korbmacher-Steiner, H.; Jäger, A.; Schauseil, M. Novel Lingual Retainer Created Using CAD/CAM Technology: Evaluation of Its Positioning Accuracy. *J. Orofac. Orthop. Fortschr. Kieferorthopadie Organ Off. J. Dtsch. Ges. Kieferorthopadie* **2015**, *76*, 164–174. [CrossRef]

38. Kravitz, N.D.; Grauer, D.; Schumacher, P.; Jo, Y. Memotain: A CAD/CAM Nickel-Titanium Lingual Retainer. *Am. J. Orthod. Dentofacial Orthop.* **2017**, *151*, 812–815. [CrossRef]

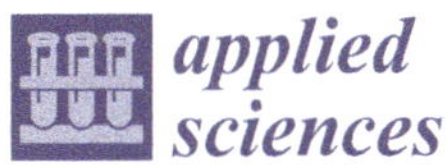

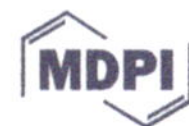

Article

The Mask Fitter, a Simple Method to Improve Medical Face Mask Adaptation Using a Customized 3D-Printed Frame during COVID-19: A Survey on Users' Acceptability in Clinical Dentistry

Alessandro Vichi [1],*, Dario Balestra [2], Cecilia Goracci [3], David R. Radford [1] and Chris Louca [1]

[1]   Dental Academy, University of Portsmouth, Portsmouth PO1 2QG, UK
[2]   School of Dentistry, Universidad Alfonso X el Sabio (UAX), Villanueva de la Canada, 28691 Madrid, Spain
[3]   Department of Medical Biotechnologies, University of Siena, 53100 Siena, Italy
*   Correspondence: alessandro.vichi@port.ac.uk; Tel.: +39-0564-25384

Featured Application: The paper shows the procedure for producing a customized low-cost "Mask Fitter" made with a tablet-based 3D-face-scan and 3D-printing that could improve the sealing of FFP2 respirators.

Abstract: COVID-19 has deeply impacted clinical strategies in dentistry and the use of surgical masks and respirators has become critical. They should adapt to the person's facial anatomy, but this is not always easy to achieve. Bellus3D Company proposed to apply their face scan software, used with selected smartphones and tablets, to design and 3D-print a bespoke "Mask Fitter" to improve the sealing of surgical masks and respirators. Twenty dental staff participants were face scanned and a Mask Fitter for FFP2 respirators was designed and 3D-printed. Participants were asked to wear their Mask Fitter over one week and then completed a survey. Questions were asked about wearing comfort, sealing confidence, glasses or loupes fogging, both with and without the Mask Fitter. Dental staff gave positive feedback, with levels of comfort during daily use reported as similar with and without the Mask Fitter; and a higher confidence in achieving a proper seal, ranging from a 10% confidence rating of a proper seal without the Mask Fitter to 75% with the Mask Fitter. Moreover, fogging problems decreased considerably. The tested Mask Fitter device could represent an easy and low-cost procedure to improve the facial adaptation of the FFP2 respirator.

Keywords: 3D-face-scanning; 3D-printing; surgical mask; FFP2 respirator; mask fitter

Citation: Vichi, A.; Balestra, D.; Goracci, C.; Radford, D.R.; Louca, C. The Mask Fitter, a Simple Method to Improve Medical Face Mask Adaptation Using a Customized 3D-Printed Frame during COVID-19: A Survey on Users' Acceptability in Clinical Dentistry . *Appl. Sci.* **2022** , *12* , 8921 . https://doi.org/10.3390/app12178921

Academic Editors: Giuseppe Andreoni and Gianluca Gambarini

Received: 29 March 2022
Accepted: 2 September 2022
Published: 5 September 2022

Publisher's Note: MDPI stays neutral with regard to jurisdictional claims in published maps and institutional affiliations.

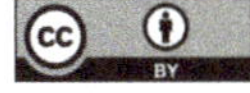

1. Introduction

After a report at the end of 2019 of unclear cases of pneumonia from China, in early 2020 the World Health Organization (WHO) declared the discovery of a new coronavirus, officially named SARS-CoV-2, with the resulting respiratory disease named COVID-19 (coronavirus disease) [1–4]. The disease continued to rapidly spread around the world, resulting in the declaration by the WHO of a pandemic [5,6]. Several countries have experienced a rapid dispersion of COVID-19, also related to the relatively easy transmission routes [7–9]. COVID-19 transmission is reported to occur through direct inhalation of droplets, coughing and sneezing or by contact with the mucous membranes of the oral cavity, the nasal cavity and the eye [10,11]. To et al. [12] reported a high concentration of SARS-CoV-2 in the saliva of people with COVID-19. Dental professionals are highly exposed to a risk of infection due to their exposure to saliva, blood and aerosol/droplet production during most dental procedures [13–16]. Therefore, the use of personal protective equipment (PPE), including gloves, masks, protective outerwear, protective surgical glass and shields, is strongly recommended to protect the eye, oral and nasal mucosa [13]. The production of aerosols and droplets during routine dental procedures cannot be completely avoided, hence the generation of highly contaminated microbial aerosol [17,18]. PPE amongst the dental profession has become increasingly important, and use of facial masks, particularly, has also been recommended for most of the population during any kind of contact with other individuals. One of the fundamental pre-requisites of a surgical mask is its ability to properly adapt to the person's facial anatomy, creating a good seal to limit as much as possible the spread of bacteria and viruses. A good face mask seal is not always easy to achieve, especially since not all human faces allow an easy adaptation of the mask. To help address these surgical mask adaptation uncertainties, Bellus3D, a USA based company, (Bellus3D, Campbell, CA, USA) has developed a system for which a custom adapted low-cost Mask Fitter can be easily and rapidly produced. The Mask Fitter has already been reported to be potentially effective in an ophthalmology related study in which a quantitative fit test (QNFT) was performed [19]. More recently, another study still performed with a QNFT on dentists reported that the 3D printed frame fitted over a surgical mask offers advantages comparable to those offered by FFP2 respirators in terms of marginal fit. However, surgical masks do not offer the same protection in terms of filtering capacity, thus the use of surgical masks with mask fitter could be considered only as a replacement in case of a FFP2 shortage [20].

The aim of the present study was to evaluate several aspects of the use of the Mask Fitter produced and delivered to a cohort of dental staff, in general practice settings, particularly concerning low-, medium- and long-term (full day) wearability.

2. Materials and Methods

The process for the fabrication of the Mask Fitter requires a face scan, followed by the design and 3D-printing of the Mask Fitter. For a face scan process, several options are available including photogrammetry, stereophotogrammetry, laser-beam scanning and structured light scanning [21]. An easy-to-use alternative is the "face ID" system implemented in the more recent generations of smartphones and tablets. The smartphones that at present can be used are any iPhone^{TM} with a TrueDepth^{TM} camera (iPhone X onwards), or an iPad Pro^{TM} (all generations). For this survey, an iPad Pro 1st generation was used. The necessary software, Bellus3D Dental Pro, can be downloaded from the Apple store. Bellus3D Dental Pro is available as a free download for basic features offering in-app purchase for advanced functionalities. This face scan system has been reported to allow trueness and precision in a clinically acceptable range [21,22]. The design of the Mask Fitter has different options. The basic version of the Mask Fitter for a surgical mask can be generated and exported free of charge, whilst the generation of the Mask Fitter with holders' name or the FFP2 ("tall") version require payment of a USD 1.99 (USA currency) fee. After installing the software, the face scan acquisition procedure is straightforward. It consists of a voice guided procedure requiring a simple left, right, up, and down sequence of head movements (Figure 1).

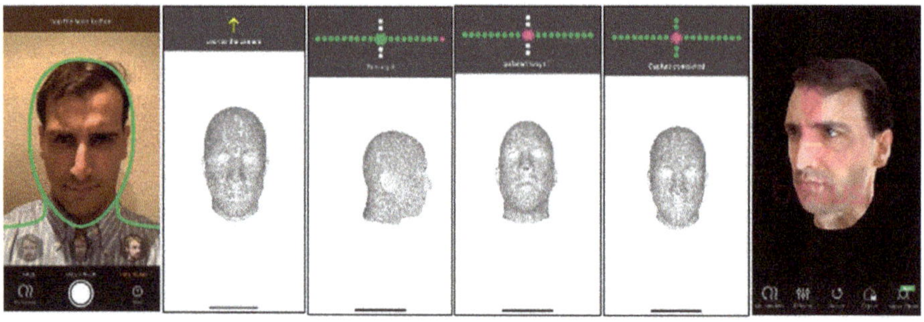

Figure 1. Face scan acquisition procedure.

Of the three available scanning options (face, face + neck, full head) the second one is recommended by the authors of the present paper for the Mask Fitter purposes. Option one (face only) takes an insufficiently detailed scan of the chin area, while option three (full head) is redundant as the back of the head is not involved in the Mask Fitter design. At the end of an approximately 30 s scan process, followed by another approximately 20 s for data computing, the 3D-representation of the face is generated. After selection of the function "mask fitting" and subsequently the selection of the desired design ("standard" for surgical masks, "tall" for FFP2), a Mask Fitter consisting of an anatomic frame is automatically designed by the software with a 10 s processing time (Figure 2a).

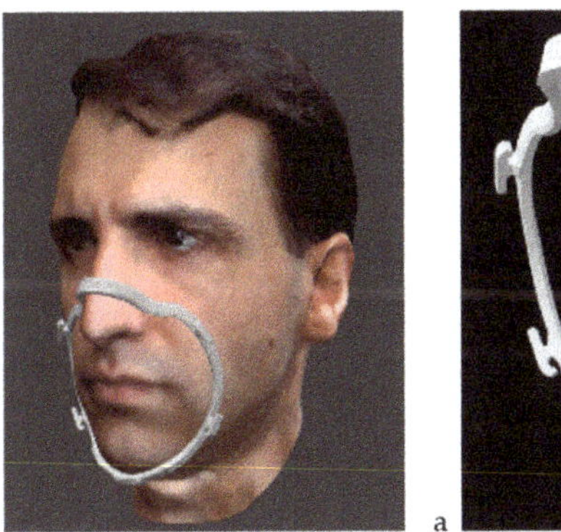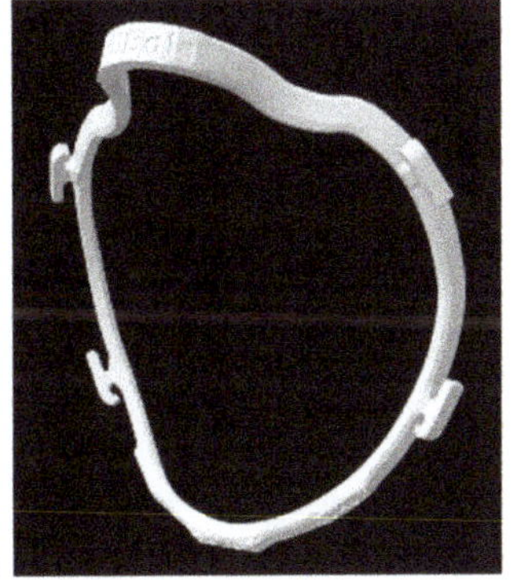

Figure 2. (**a**,**b**): The Mask Fitter design generated by the software.

The generated Mask Fitter design can then be exported as a .stl file (Figure 2b). The free version of the software does not allow the face-scanning to be saved, but it does allow the sending of the .stl file of the generated design of the Mask Fitter via email. Once the file is received by email it can be 3D-printed. Partner services are suggested from the Company itself, but any 3D-printing services, available online at different, but reasonable prices (e.g., GBP 10–15 UK currency), can be used. Alternatively, and more conveniently, the Mask Fitter can be printed by any Office, Department, University, Company, Dental Laboratory or even personal 3D-printer (Figures 3–5) as there are no special requirements for the printer and the material. A basic Stereolithography (SLA—Resin) 3D-printer or a basic Fused Deposition Modeling (FDM—filament) 3D-printer can efficiently 3D-print the Mask Fitter.

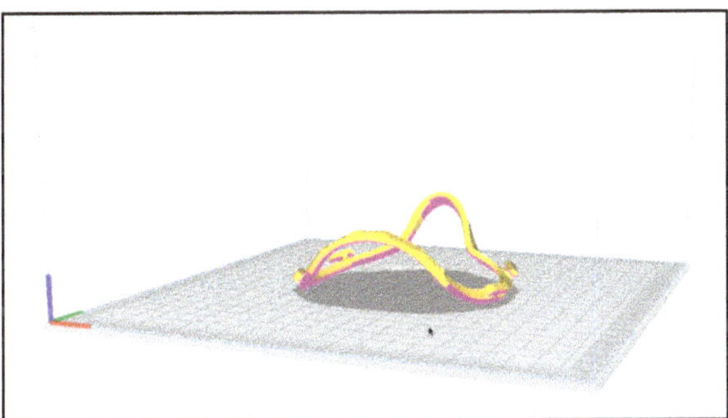

Figure 3. A GCode is generated by a 3D-printing slicing software (Ultimaker Cura).

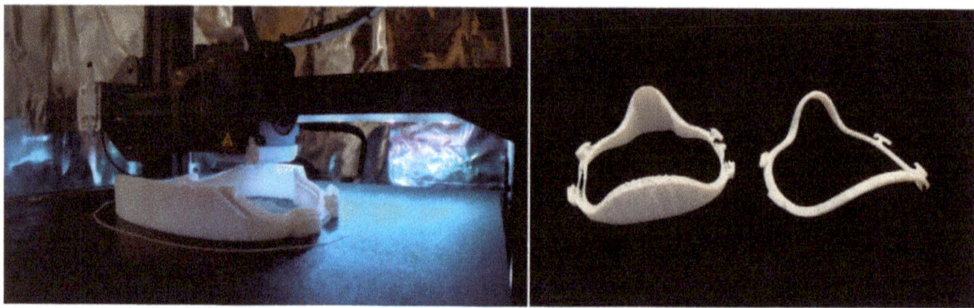

Figure 4. A 3D-printing process with a personal filament 3D-printer (left) and the Mask Fitter after printing and finishing.

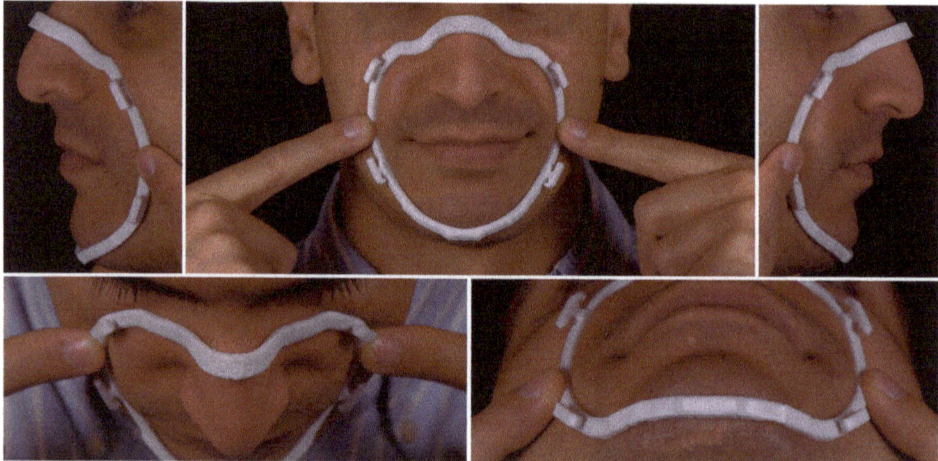

Figure 5. The Mask Fitter adaptation to the scanned face anatomy.

For the present study, a total of 20 dental staff were recruited for this service evaluation selected following "convenience sample" selection criteria, and they voluntarily agreed to try the Mask Fitter. A written consent was obtained from each of the participants, by which they agreed to participate in the study and to have their data used as part of the research. They were face-scanned and then their Mask Fitters were 3D-printed as previously described. The emailed .stl files were processed for slicing with the software Ultimaker Cura 4.7.1 (Ultimaker BV, Utrecht, The Netherlands) and 3D-printed with the printer Anycubic Mega S (Anycubic, Shenzhen, Guangdong, China) set with Generic Polylactic Acid (PLA), Profiles 0.1 mm and Infill 100%. PLA and Acrylonitrile Butadiene Styrene (ABS) are the recommended filament, but there are no specific restrictions providing the printed surfaces are not porous. PLA and ABS can be disinfected by immersion in the disinfecting solution recommended for each material. The Mask Fitter is placed on the external side of the surgical mask, and thereby does not need any special biocompatibility or antiallergic properties. For the present survey, the filament 1.75 mm PLA 3D-Printer Filament (Anycubic, Shenzhen, Guangdong, China) in grey shade, was used. This is a biodegradable filament made from lactic acid, produced via starch fermentation during corn wet milling. The available information for this material is: Diameter 1.75 ± 0.02 mm, Tensile strength ≥ 55 MPa, Hardness HRC 105–110, Density 1.25 g $\pm$ cm^3. For the present study, it has been 3D-printed with the nozzle temperature at 210 °C and printing platform at 60°.

The fitter is designed with hooks and is secured to the FFP2 mask elastic band by means of these hooks (Figure 6).

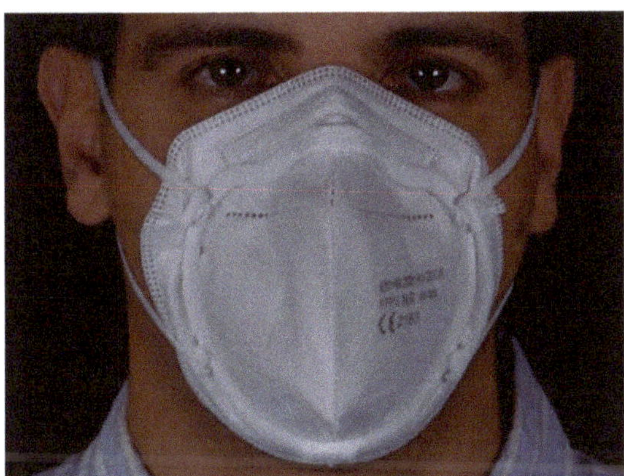

Figure 6. The Mask Fitter positioning.

After a preliminary phase designed to achieve a comfortable fit of the Mask Fitter, the subjects involved in the study were asked to wear the FFP2 for: (i) 1 h (short-term use, simulating a single patient treatment time); (ii) 4 h (mid-term use, simulating half-day work); and (iii) 8 h (simulating full-day work), with and without the Mask Fitter. A Google form survey was designed with 27 questions. The 20 dental staff were invited to complete the survey in order to provide a preliminary report on some aspects of PPE use, and on the acceptance and first impressions of its daily use.

3. Results

The survey and its results are reported in Table 1 (Demographic data); Table 2 (Prior to COVID-19); Table 3 (After COVID-19); Table 4 (The Mask Fitter); Table 5 (Fogging). Numbers refer to the relative question of the survey. Responses were received from all the participants (20).

Table 1. Section 1: Demographic data.

	Demographic Data			
1. Age	20–29	30–39	40–49	50+
	0 (0%)	6 (30%)	5 (25%)	9 (45%)
2. Gender	Male	Female	Non-binary	Prefer not to say
	5 (25%)	15 (75%)	0 (0%)	0 (0%)
3. Qualification	Dentist	Dental Nurse	Dental Hygienist	Other
	7 (35%)	11 (55%)	2 (10%)	0 (0%)

Table 2. Section 2: Prior to COVID-19.

Prior to COVID-19			
4. Prior to COVID-19 did you routinely wear a face mask?			
Yes	No		
19 (95%)	1 (5%)		
5. If you wore a mask was it:			
All the time	Only for contact with patients	Only for treating patients	Only for aerosol generating procedures
5 (25%)	4 (20%)	7 (35%)	4 (20%)

6. What type of mask was it? (more than one choice allowed)				
Simple face mask (e.g., acrylic screen)	Surgical face mask	FFP2	FFP3	other
9 (45%)	20 (100%)	0 (0%)	0 (0%)	1 (5%)

7. For how many years have you been wearing a mask of any type?			
0–5	6–10	11–20	20+
3 (15%)	2 (10%)	7 (35%)	8 (40%)

Table 3. Section 3: After COVID-19.

After COVID-19				
8. What type of face mask do you currently use? (more than one choice allowed)				
Simple Face Mask (e.g., Acrylic Screen)	Surgical Face Mask	FFP2	FFP3	Other
17 (85%)	10 (50%)	20 (100%)	1 (5%)	2 (10%)
9. How easy is it to achieve a comfortable fit of your mask on your face?				
Very easy	Easy	Medium	Difficult	Very difficult
0 (0%)	0 (0%)	4 (20%)	5 (25%)	11 (55%)
10. Over short-term use (up to one hour) how comfortable is your mask?				
Very low	Low	Medium	High	Very high
0 (0%)	0 (0%)	9 (45%)	6 (30%)	0 (0%)
11. Over mid-term use (up to four hours) how comfortable is your mask?				
Very low	Low	Medium	High	Very high
0 (0%)	3 (15%)	11 (55%)	6 (30%)	5 (25%)
12. Over long-term use (full working day) how comfortable is your mask?				
Very low	Low	Medium	High	Very high
3 (15%)	9 (45%)	6 (30%)	2 (10%)	0 (0%)
13. How confident are you that you have achieved an effective seal?				
Very low	Low	Medium	High	Very high
0 (0%)	3 (15%)	8 (40%)	7 (35%)	2 (10%)
14. Do you think that a customized face mask adapted to you face anatomy would be beneficial?				
Yes	No	Do not know		
15 (75%)	1 (5%)	4 (20%)		

Table 4. Section 4: The Mask Fitter.

The Mask Fitter				
15. How easy is it to achieve a comfortable fit of the Mask Fitter on your face?				
Very low	Low	Medium	High	Very high
2 (10%)	1 (5%)	5 (25%)	7 (35%)	5 (25%)
16. Over short-term use (up to one hour) how comfortable is your Mask Fitter?				
Very low	Low	Medium	High	Very high
2 (10%)	2 (10%)	6 (30%)	6 (30%)	4 (20%)
17. Over mid-term use (up to four hours) how comfortable is your Mask Fitter?				
Very low	Low	Medium	High	Very high
2 (10%)	5 (25%)	8 (40%)	6 (30%)	2 (10%)
18. Over long-term use (up to eight hours) how comfortable is your Mask Fitter?				
Very low	Low	Medium	High	Very high
5 (25%)	8 (40%)	5 (25%)	2 (10%)	0 (0%)
19. How confident are you that you have achieved an effective seal with the Mask Fitter?				
Very low	Low	Medium	High	Very high
0 (0%)	1 (5%)	1 (5%)	3 (15%)	15 (75%)
20. How would you rate the cleaning procedure for the Mask Fitter?				
Very difficult	Difficult	Medium	Easy	Very easy
0 (0%)	0 (0%)	1 (5%)	4 (20%)	15 (75%)
21. Would you routinely use the Mask Fitter to improve the FFP2 seal?				
Yes	Only for selected patients	Only for selected procedures (aerosol-generating)	For both selected patients and procedures	No
5 (25%)	0 (0%)	3 (15%)	10 (50%)	2 (10%)

Table 5. Section 5: Fogging.

Fogging				
23. Do you wear loupes?				
Yes	No			
3 (15%)	17 (85%)			
24. Do you wear glasses?				
Yes	No			
13 (65%)	7 (35%)			
25. Is loupes or glasses fogging a problem when wearing FFP2 without Mask Fitter? (only for those answering yes to either question 22 or 23)				
Very low	Low	Medium	High	Very high
1 (6.7%)	3 (20%)	4 (26.7%)	5 (33.3%)	2 (13.3%)
26. Is loupes or glasses fogging a problem when wearing FFP2 with the Mask Fitter? (only for those answering yes to either question 22 or 23)				
Very low	Low	Medium	High	Very high
6 (40%)	5 (33.3%)	3 (20%)	0 (0%)	1 (6.7%)

22. Can you please give the reason (for your answer to question 21)?

18 responses received.

The comments broadly followed the response to question 21, "for both selected patients and procedures" and "positive comments".

For both selected patients and procedures

Wearing all the time is heavy but for selected procedures and patients it is fine.

Breathing is anyway more difficult and without it, thus I would say that selected patients and procedures would be better.

Positive comments

Better seal and no fogging on screen even when used for a long time.

I have a thin face and all the masks (with the only exception of 3 M Aura which is a FFP3) have sealing problems.

Better seal thus better protection.

A final overall comment was posed to the participants

27. Any other comments that you have regarding face masks or Mask Fitter

12 responses which centred on pressure on the nose.

Nose is a little compressed.

Easier to fit than the other protections. Nose is a problem because my glasses and my screen go on the nose, thus the position of the filter (on the nose) is not "free" and gives some pain after hours of use.

The fitting is never perfect. Without elastic bands it creates problems for the ears. With the elastic bands it creates problems to the nose and chin.

4. Discussion

It is known that FFP2 masks can provide an efficient filter against droplets responsible for the transmission of the COVID-19 infection. The more the FFP2 is securely adapted to the face, the better the seal, thereby preventing the spread of infection. Fit testing is mandatory in some countries e.g., in the United Kingdom and has been employed to ensure masks (FFP2 and FFP3) fit adequately to ensure a good seal for people working in public health systems.

In dentistry, great attention has been directed towards Aerosol Generating Procedures (AGP) such as ultrasonic scaling and use of a high-speed air turbine handpiece with water. During these procedures, aerosols are generated, and the possibility to be infected is high. The "Mask Fitter" is an attempt to help dental professionals wearing masks in clinical environments to improve the seal of the mask.

Concerning the Survey, Section 1, questions 1, 2 and 3 reported demographic data. Of the 20 dental staff participants, 30% were aged 30–39 years, 45% were aged 40–49 years and 55% were 50+ years old; and 75% were female. The dental staff comprised Dentists 35%, Hygienists 10%, and Dental Nurses 55%. The dental staff who participated in the study came from 4 different general dental practices.

Section 2 concerned the use of PPE prior to the COVID-19 pandemic. In question 4, 95% of the dental staff declared that they already routinely used a protection system with only one exception. All of the dental staff used the surgical face mask, 45% a shield with or without the surgical mask. In question 5, before COVID-19, 20% wore a mask all the time, another 20% only when having clinical contact with patients, 35% when treating patients and only 25% wore a mask all the time. As expected, the situation changed substantially after the COVID-19 health emergency (Section 3).

Dental staff declared the use of a wide range of protection, with FFP2 adopted by 100% of the participants. Face shields were also widely used in combination with FFP2 masks. Surgical masks were still used but mostly overlaying the FFP2 as an additional layer of protection, with a view to replacing the surgical mask between patients, retaining the FFP2 mask which has a higher cost and at least early in the pandemic were much harder to source. Only one operator reported using a FFP3 mask (with valve and surgical mask overlying) and 2 reported using alternative systems such as an open helmet and special glasses resembling a scuba diver mask, both used with FFP2.

Fitting and ease of use of the FFP2 (question 9) was reported to be medium to very high for all the staff members involved, showing that this PPE is now routinely used in daily practice. However, the wearing of FFP2 masks is considered to be tiring. In questions 10, 11 and 12 dental staff reported that wearing the mask is comfortable for up to 1 h (rating 3, 4 or 5 out of 5), reducing between 1 to 4 h (rating 2, 3 and 4 out of 5), and further reduced comfort over a full day of use (rating 1 to 4 out of 5 with 45% rating 2).

Confidence in obtaining a proper seal (question 13) was widely reported, with 15% rating 2 out of 5, 40% rating 3, 35% rating 4 and only 2% rating 5 out of 5. This means that dental staff were wearing the FFP2, but they still had some concerns regarding its efficacy. Interest in a system designed to improve this efficacy (question 14) was 75% with only 1 staff member answering no (Figure 7).

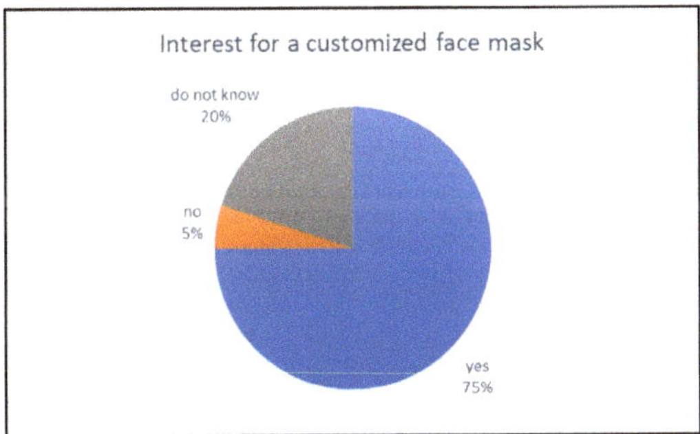

Figure 7. Interest for a customized device.

Section 4 evaluated the Mask Fitter.

Concerning the ease of wearing the Mask Fitter (question 15), the outcome was widespread, with 10% of dental staff rating 1 out of 5, 5% rating 2, 25% rating 3, 35% rating 4 and 25% rating 5. In total 85% rated the ease of wearing from medium to very high.

Wearing (questions 16, 17 and 18) was reported to be comfortable over time, within one hour (3 out of 5 for 30%, 4 for 30%, 5 for 20%). The percentage decreased when worn 1 to 4 h, as well as all day long, with only 10% still rating 4 and no one rating 5 at the end of the working day.

Interestingly, even if slightly differently distributed, the percentage from medium to very high levels of comfort at the end of the day were globally very similar both without and with the Mask Fitter (respectively 40% and 35%), showing a good acceptance of this extra item (Figure 8).

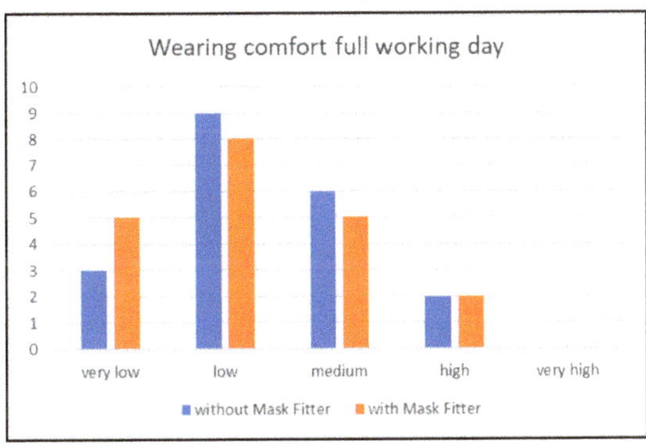

Figure 8. Wearing comfort over full working day, without and with Mask Fitter.

A remarkable outcome from this service evaluation was question 19 where dental staff declared, when wearing the Mask Fitter, to have reached a higher confidence on obtaining a proper seal with 75% rating 5 out of 5. The difference with the same data without the Mask Fitter (only 10% rating 5 out of 5) was impressive (Figure 9).

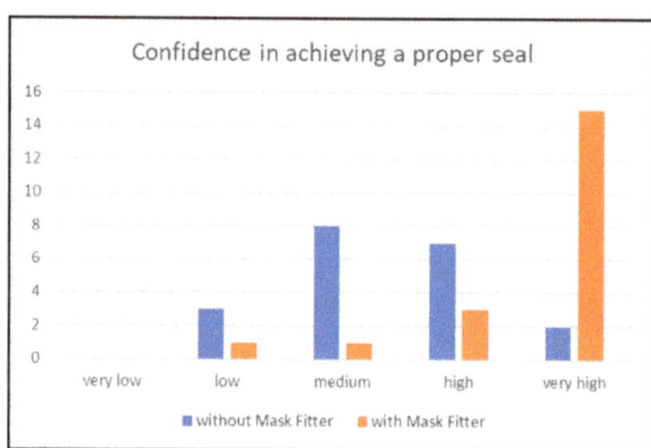

Figure 9. Confidence in achieving an appropriate seal with and without Mask Fitter.

In question 20, 75% of the dental staff rated 5 out of 5 the ease of cleaning the face mask (performed by immersion in disinfectant). When asked (question 21) if they would introduce the Mask Fitter routinely, 25% of the staff stated that they would use it all the time, while 65 % declared that they would use it for selected patients, or procedures, or both. Only 10% reported that they would not use the Mask Fitter (Figure 10).

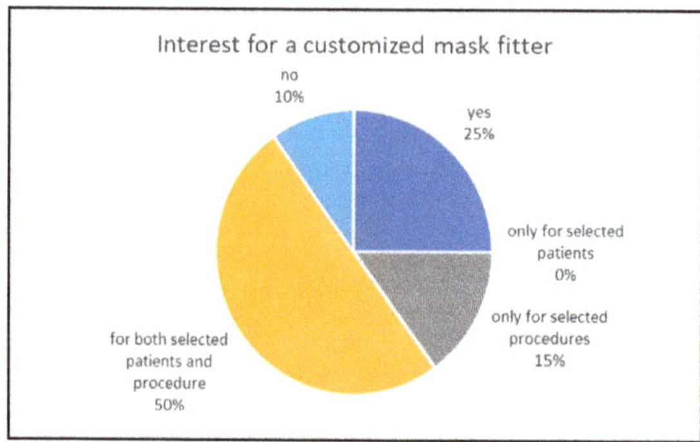

Figure 10. Interest in wearing the Mask Fitter routinely.

Question (22) invited free text feedback from the participants on the reasons for their responses to question 21. The reasons for not adopting the routine use of the Mask Fitter were that people feel sufficiently safe with the FFP2 alone. The most frequent reason for not adopting the Mask Fitter for continuous use, but more likely for patients and/or selected procedures, was that wearing the Mask Fitter all the time was tiring. Therefore, its use for limited situations such as aerosol generating procedures or for those occasions when patients declare no symptoms at the COVID-19 triage stage, with the absence of a fever, but there may be some uncertainty due to a sporadic cough and/or the need to occasionally blow their nose, might be the appropriate indication for the Mask Fitter.

Section 5 focused on the effect of wearing the Mask Fitter on the fogging of glasses or loupes. From questions 23 and 24 it was reported that only 15% of the participants used loupes, while 65% wore glasses. A total of 25% of the participants wore neither loupes nor glasses, thus they did not answer the following two questions (25 and 26). Even if the distribution of the fifteen answers related to fogging was quite widespread, the effect of the Mask Fitter looked beneficial. Without the Mask Fitter (question 25), the participants reported a total of 73% medium (3 out of 5) to very high (5 of 5) fogging problems, that decreased to a total of 27% (question 26) when wearing the Mask Fitter, thus showing a high capability to reduce fogging problems (Figure 11).

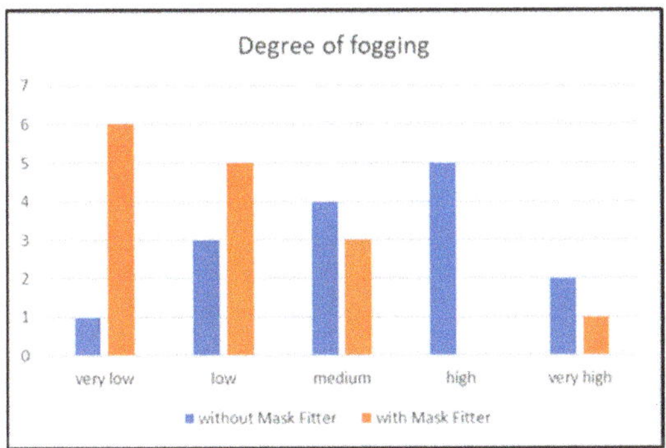

Figure 11. Effects of Mask Fitter on fogging of loupes and glasses.

The last question of the survey (question 27) invited free text answers on the use of the Mask Fitter. There were some reported problems in obtaining the proper adaptation using a trial-and-error procedure for obtaining an appropriate tightening with or without the use of an additional rubber band on the back of the head. Staff reported that once a good adaptation was obtained, it was easy to be reproduced when worn again. They commented on a sense of constriction on the nose and consequent oral breathing. Some participants reported that due to the position of the nasal arch, even light pressure immediately made it difficult to breathe through the nose. This might be due to a possible slight deformation on the face scan in the nasal area, as reported by Alisha et al. [23]. Participants generally agreed that this is the main aspect requiring improvement, even if none of the participants reported any sores and/or scars. The authors of the present paper consider proposing to the Company an optional function to be implemented in the software that could allow to "lift" the nose arch by a small amount, e.g., 0.5, 1.0, 1.5, 2.0 mm, both in the vertical and lateral dimension, to improve the wearability of the Mask Fitter, reducing the pressure on the nose. Alternatively, the application of a patch on the nose before face-scanning is another possible option to investigate. Another alternative that can be explored is the 3D-printing of polymers less rigid than the PLA used in the present study, like Polyethylene Terephthalate Glycol-modified (PETG), Thermoplastic Polyurethane (TPU) or Thermoplastic Elastomer (TPE). Further research is also required to categorize the variations in facial anatomy, which may explain the differences in comfort reported. A further study is in progress aimed at evaluating whether dental staff tested for mask sealing efficacy, and not passing the test, could have a beneficial effect from the use of the Mask Fitter. In the future, the use of different three-dimensional digitation technologies, or virtualization, reverse engineering and development of numerical methods could also be evaluated.

5. Conclusions

Dental staff using the bespoke Mask Fitter reported positively, with levels of comfort during daily use comparable with and without the Mask Fitter. Moreover, a much higher confidence in achieving a proper seal was reported. Moreover, fogging problems decreased considerably. Based on this preliminary survey, it can be concluded that the Mask Fitter device designed by Bellus3D received a good acceptance by Dental staff and therefore could represent an easy, low-cost procedure to improve the adaptation of the FFP2 mask.

Author Contributions: Conceptualization, A.V. and C.L.; methodology, A.V. and D.R.R.; software, D.B.; investigation, A.V.; data curation, C.G.; writing—original draft preparation, A.V.; writing—review and editing, C.G., D.R.R. and C.L. visualization, D.B. All authors have read and agreed to the published version of the manuscript.

Funding: This research received no external funding.

Institutional Review Board Statement: The study was conducted according to the guidelines of the Declaration of Helsinki and approved by the Institutional Review Board of of the National Board of Dentist (FNOMCeO—CAO) (protocol n. 369 of 8.2.2022).

Informed Consent Statement: Informed consent was obtained from all subjects involved in the study.

Data Availability Statement: The data presented in this study are available on request from the corresponding author. The data are not publicly available due to the university policy on access.

Acknowledgments: The authors are thankful to the owners and staff of the dental surgeries of Cecilia Goracci, Fabio Pallari, Raffaello Trusendi and Francesco Deodato, and Alessandro Vichi for their willingness to participate in the study.

Conflicts of Interest: The authors declare no conflict of interest.

References

1. Lu, R.; Zhao, X.; Li, J.; Niu, P.; Yang, B.; Wu, H.; Wang, W.; Song, H.; Huang, B.; Zhu, N.; et al. Genomic characterization and epidemiology of 2019 novel coronavirus: Implications for virus origins and receptor binding. *Lancet* **2020**, *395*, 565–574. [PubMed]
2. Wang, D.; Hu, B.; Hu, C.; Zhu, F.; Liu, X.; Zhang, J.; Wang, B.; Xiang, H.; Cheng, Z.; Xiong, Y.; et al. Clinical characteristics of 138 hospitalized patients with 2019 novel coronavirus-infected pneumonia in Wuhan, China. *JAMA* **2020**, *323*, 1061–1069. [CrossRef] [PubMed]
3. Yang, Y.; Lu, Q.; Liu, M.; Wang, Y.; Zhang, A.; Jalali, N.; Dean, N.; Longini, I.; Halloran, M.E.; Xu, B.; et al. Epidemiological and clinical features of the 2019 novel coronavirus outbreak in China. *medRxiv* 2020. [CrossRef]
4. Yang, Y.; Peng, F.; Wang, R.; Guan, K.; Jiang, T.; Xu, G.; Sun, J.; Chang, C. The deadly coronaviruses: The 2003 SARS pandemic and the 2020 novel coronavirus epidemic in China. *J. Autoimmun.* **2020**, *109*, 102434. [CrossRef]
5. Backer, J.A.; Klinkenberg, D.; Wallinga, J. Incubation period of 2019 novel coronavirus (2019-nCoV) infections among travelers from Wuhan, China, 20–28 January. *Euro. Surveill.* **2020**, *25*, 2000062. [CrossRef]
6. Mahase, E. China coronavirus: WHO declares international emergency as death toll exceeds 200. *BMJ* **2020**, *368*, m408. [CrossRef]
7. Chen, N.; Zhou, M.; Dong, X.; Qu, J.; Gong, F.; Han, Y.; Qiu, Y.; Wang, J.; Liu, Y.; Wei, Y.; et al. Epidemiological and clinical characteristics of 99 cases of 2019 novel coronavirus pneumonia in Wuhan, China: A descriptive study. *Lancet* **2020**, *395*, 507–513.
8. Chen, J. Pathogenicity and transmissibility of 2019-nCoV—A quick overview and comparison with other emerging viruses. *Microb. Infect.* **2020**, *22*, 69–71.
9. Rothe, C.; Schunk, M.; Sothmann, P.; Bretzel, G.; Froeschl, G.; Wallrauch, C.; Zimmer, T.; Thiel, V.; Janke, C.; Guggemos, W.; et al. Transmission of 2019-nCoV infection from an asymptomatic contact in Germany. *N. Engl. J. Med.* **2020**, *382*, 970–971.
10. Kampf, G.; Todt, D.; Pfaender, S.; Steinmann, E. Persistence of coronaviruses on inanimate surfaces and its inactivation with biocidal agents. *J. Hosp. Infect.* **2020**, *104*, 246–251.
11. Lu, C.W.; Liu, X.F.; Jia, Z.F. 2019-nCoV transmission through the ocular surface must not be ignored. *Lancet* **2020**, *395*, e39.
12. To, K.K.; Tsang, O.T.; Yip, C.C.-Y.; Chan, K.H.; Wu, T.C.; Chan, J.M.C.; Leung, W.S.; Chik, T.S.; Choi, C.Y.; Kandamby, D.H.; et al. Consistent detection of 2019 novel coronavirus in saliva. *Clin. Infect. Dis.* **2020**, *71*, 841–843. [CrossRef]
13. Meng, L.; Hua, F.; Bian, Z. Coronavirus disease 2019 (COVID-19): Emerging and future challenges for dental and oral medicine. *J. Dent. Res.* **2020**, *99*, 481–487. [CrossRef]
14. Peng, X.; Xu, X.; Li, Y.; Cheng, L.; Zhou, X.; Ren, B. Transmission routes of 2019-nCoV and controls in dental practice. *Int. J. Oral Sci.* **2020**, *12*, 9. [PubMed]
15. Xu, H.; Zhong, L.; Deng, J.; Peng, J.; Dan, H.; Zeng, X.; Li, T.; Chen, Q. High expression of ACE2 receptor of 2019-nCoV on the epithelial cells of oral mucosa. *Int. J. Oral. Sci.* **2020**, *12*, 8. [PubMed]
16. van Doremalen, N.; Bushmaker, T.; Morris, D.H.; Holbrook, M.G.; Gamble, A.; Williamson, B.N.; Tamin, A.; Harcourt, J.L.; Thornburg, N.J.; Gerber, S.I.; et al. Aerosol and surface stability of SARS-CoV-2 as compared with SARS-CoV-1. *N. Engl. J. Med.* **2020**, *382*, 1564–1567. [CrossRef] [PubMed]
17. Helmis, C.G.; Tzoutzas, J.; Flocas, H.A.; Halios, C.H.; Stathopoulou, O.I.; Assimakopoulos, V.D.; Panis, V.; Apostolatou, M.; Sgouros, G.; Adam, E. Indoor air quality in a dentistry clinic. *Sci. Total Environ.* **2007**, *377*, 349–365.
18. Sebastiani, F.R.; Dym, H.; Kirpalani, T. Infection control in the dental office. *Dent. Clin. N. Am.* **2017**, *61*, 435–457.
19. Liu, J.; Ma, J.; Ahmed, I.I.K.; Varma, D.K. Effectiveness of a 3D-printed mask fitter in an ophthalmology setting during COVID-19. *Can. J. Ophthalmol.* **2022**, *57*, 161–166. [CrossRef]
20. Kongkiatkamon, S.; Wongkornchaowalit, N.; Kiatthanakorn, Y.; Tonphu, S.; Kunanusont, C. Quantitative Fit Test of a 3D Printed Frame Fitted Over a Surgical Mask: An Alternative Option to N95 Respirator. *Int. J. Dent.* **2022**, *2022*, 1270106. [CrossRef]

21. Piedra-Cascón, W.; Meyer, J.M.; Methani, M.M.; Revilla-León, M. Accuracy (trueness and precision) of a dual-structured light facial scanner and interexaminer reliability. *J. Prosthet. Dent.* **2020**, *124*, 567–574. [CrossRef] [PubMed]
22. da Silva Marques, D.N.; Aparício Aguiar Alves, R.V.; Marques Pinto, R.J.; Bártolo Caramês, J.R.; de Oliveira Francisco, H.C.; Mendez Caramês, J.M. Facial scanner accuracy with different superimposition methods—In vivo study. *Int. J. Prosthodont.* **2021**, *34*, 578–584. [CrossRef] [PubMed]
23. Alisha, K.H.; Batra, P.; Raghavan, S.; Sharma, K.; Talwar, A. A new frame for orienting infants with cleft lip and palate during 3-Dimensional facial scanning. *Cleft Palate Craniofac. J.* **2021**, *59*, 946–950. [CrossRef] [PubMed]

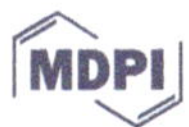

Article

3D-Printed Teeth with Multicolored Layers as a Tool for Evaluating Cavity Preparation by Dental Students

Diva Lugassy [1,2], Mohamed Awad [3], Asaf Shely [3], Moshe Davidovitch [2], Raphael Pilo [1] and Tamar Brosh [1,*]

[1] Department of Oral Biology, The Maurice and Gabriela Goldschleger School of Dental Medicine, Sackler Faculty of Medicine, Tel Aviv University, Tel Aviv 6997801, Israel; diva_lugassy@hotmail.com (D.L.); rafipilo@tauex.tau.ac.il (R.P.)

[2] Department of Orthodontics, The Maurice and Gabriela Goldschleger School of Dental Medicine, Sackler Faculty of Medicine, Tel Aviv University, Tel Aviv 6997801, Israel; moshedavidovitch@gmail.com

[3] Department of Oral Rehabilitation, The Maurice and Gabriela Goldschleger School of Dental Medicine, Sackler Faculty of Medicine, Tel Aviv University, Tel Aviv 6997801, Israel; k.awad007@gmail.com (M.A.); asafshely@gmail.com (A.S.)

* Correspondence: tbrosh@tauex.tau.ac.il; Tel.: +972-52-2777033; Fax: +972-3-6409250

Abstract: Accurate assessment of dental student performance during preclinical operative mannequin courses is an essential milestone within the educational process. Training on novel, multicolored 3D-printed teeth resulted in higher performances of the students in comparison to training on standard, monochromatic plastic teeth. However, low reliability of students' grading using standard, monochromatic plastic teeth was reported. The aim of this study was to verify whether the use of 3D multicolored teeth can (1) provide better inter- and intra-examiner reliability, and (2) assess the effect of instructors' experience on their reliability. The novel tooth analogs consisted of digitally planned and 3D-printed plastic teeth containing green, yellow, and red stratifications according to increasing depths of preparation. Thirty-seven dental students performed three Class I preparations on the 3D-printed teeth, and these underwent blind evaluation by two examiners of varied experience at two timepoints. The data were compared with preparations done on conventional (monochromatic) plastic teeth. Results indicated excellent inter-examiner reliability on 3D-printed teeth ($0.768 < \text{ICC} < 0.929$), but only moderate reliability with conventional plastic teeth ($0.314 < \text{ICC} < 0.672$). The examiner having more experience was found to show higher intra-examiner reliability (ICC = 0.716 and 0.612 using 3D-printed teeth and conventional teeth, respectively) than the less experienced examiner (ICC = 0.481 and 0.095 using 3D-printed teeth and conventional teeth, respectively). The novel, multicolored 3D-printed teeth can provide more objective evaluation of cavity preparation compared with conventional plastic teeth.

Keywords: dental students; cavity preparation; 3D-printed teeth; teachers' evaluation

Citation: Lugassy, D.; Awad, M.; Shely, A.; Davidovitch, M.; Pilo, R.; Brosh, T. 3D-Printed Teeth with Multicolored Layers as a Tool for Evaluating Cavity Preparation by Dental Students. *Appl. Sci.* **2021**, *11*, 6406. https://doi.org/10.3390/app11146406

Academic Editor: Kathrin Becker

Received: 24 May 2021
Accepted: 28 June 2021
Published: 12 July 2021

1. Introduction

Dentistry is a medical profession that requires fine motor skills [1], hand–eye coordination [2], and exceptional spatial perception [3]. Furthermore, perceptual learning is needed in order to develop indirect visualization using a mirror [4,5]. These prerequisites have led dental educators to develop simulators in order to assist in the teaching of these skills [6].

The dental mannequin is the traditional simulator used to prepare dental students for treating patients; it is an anatomic construction of a human head and jaws containing plastic duplicates of each tooth arranged in a normal occlusion, on which the novice dental student is taught to perform basic dental procedures. Dental students have been shown to be particularly stressed during their preclinical studies [7]—more so when being taught cavity preparations and endodontic treatment [8]. Evaluating student performance under these conditions is further complicated because of poor examiner reliability due to human subjectivity, compounded by a paucity of objective parameters. Studies have shown that the conventional clinical evaluating systems—"glance and grade", which provides an overall mark; and the "analytical method", which utilizes specific criteria and checklists—have low reliability and validity due to high inter- and intra-examiner variability [9–11]. Sharaf et al. (2007) [9] concluded that both evaluation methods showed disagreement and high variability between examiners regarding the evaluation of operative dental procedures on plastic teeth. Jenkins et al. (1996) [10] demonstrated that instructors grading preclinical operative procedures using a glance and grade method have a high degree of inter-examiner variability, and highlighted the need for a more comprehensive system of assessing preclinical performance. Salvendy et al. (1973) [12] found not only inter-examiner variability, but also wide intra-examiner variation when the same instructor evaluated the same cavity preparation on a second occasion.

These realizations, coupled with applied digital technologies, have prompted the development of more objective and reliable methods of teaching and evaluating outcomes [13–15]. For example, PrepCheck (Dentsply Sirona, Wals, Austria) makes use of CAD/CAM (computer-assisted design and computer-assisted manufacturing) technology by comparing scans of cavity preparations with a standardized "master" preparation [16]. In addition, the Dental Teacher system (KaVo Dental, Biberach, Germany) includes a 3D scanner, PC, and three software modules for preparation validation [15].

Studies of these newer methods of evaluation have shown them to be more effective than traditional methods, primarily in self-assessment and self-directed learning of manual skills [14]. Other studies have deduced that these methods do not improve student comprehension of the skills, because of the unrealistic goal of manually reproducing any preparation exactly according to predefined values [15,17]. Therefore, obtaining an objective perspective for preparation evaluation remains a challenge.

An attempt to attain this goal using a novel, 3D-printed tooth model composed of multicolored layers was recently introduced [18]. This 3D multicolored tooth model, replacing the monocolored standard plastic teeth, was shown to be effective in the self-learning of dental students during the process of acquiring new manual skills [18]. It was concluded that this unique design provides real-time augmented visual feedback during the teaching exercise [18]. Therefore, it was assumed that the color scheme will make students' preparation evaluation by clinical instructors more objective, which could potentially reduce inter- and intra-examiner variability.

The aims of the present study were (1) to compare students' clinical assessment of cavity preparations using the multicolored 3D model to the conventional plastic teeth by evaluating inter- and intra-examiner variability, and (2) to evaluate the effect of instructors' clinical experience on the reliability of their evaluations of clinical performance.

2. Materials and Methods

2.1. Participants

Thirty-seven dental students (20 females, 17 males, mean age 25.7 ± 1.81 years, range 23–29 years) in the 2018 academic year participated in the present study. The dental students were in their fourth (15 students, mean age 25.2 ± 1.94 years), fifth (10 students, mean age 25.7 ± 2.11 years), and sixth (12 students, mean age 26.5 ± 1.16 years) years of dentistry studies on a six-year program. All participants signed informed consent approved by the Ethics Committee of Tel Aviv University.

2.2. Dental Training Models

2.2.1. Conventional Plastic Teeth

(Figure 1): Typically, dental students acquire manual dexterity by practicing on replicas of human teeth formed from plastic material (Nissin Dental Products Inc., Nakagoku, Japan) arranged within a mannequin head (Columbia, Dentalez, Malvern, PA, USA model AH-1-BP), which acts as a simulation of clinical conditions. These plastic teeth are made of a single acrylic resin material and are of a single homogeneous color (ivory), and simulate arch traits (maxilla or mandible) and type traits (anatomically correct crown shapes of each tooth).

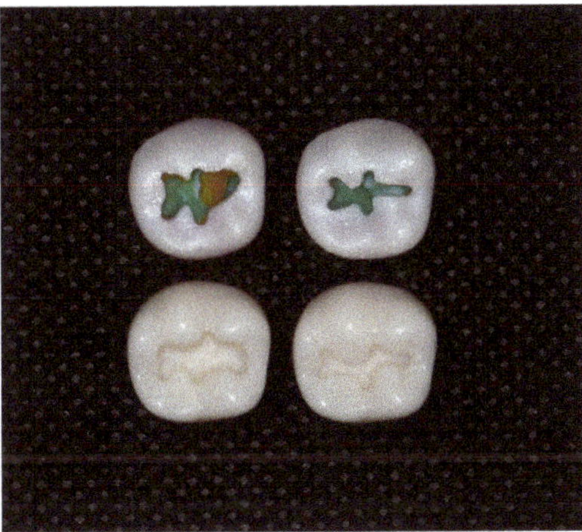

Figure 1. Upper row: Class I preparations in 3D-printed teeth with multicolored layers. Lower row: Class I preparation in conventional plastic teeth. Left column: preparations that are too wide and deep. Right column: ideal preparations.

2.2.2. 3D-Printed Teeth with Multicolored Layers

(Figure 1): The analog models of regular plastic teeth described above were digitally scanned using an Einscan-SP 3D Scanner (Shining 3D®, Hangzhou, China), the files of which were uploaded into FUSION 360 CAD/CAM 2017 software 3D-Builder programs (AUTODESK, San Rafael, CA, USA) and MySolidWorks 2017–2018 (SOLIDWORKS, Waltham, MA, USA), intended for planning models for 3D printing. After attaining the Standard Tessellation Language (STL) files, a master model of each tooth—containing multicolored layers analogous to the traffic light array (i.e., green, yellow, and red) as internal layers—was designed for each tooth. The precise outer/enveloping layers, as well as the cavity preparation of each model (both in white color), were planned according to specific wall forms, depths, and marginal forms, owing to the principles of ideal cavity preparation for amalgam restoration.

The design for the tooth model was planned for Class I cavity preparation, according to Black's classification [19], as if for an amalgam restoration including central fossa and pits and fissures on the occlusal surface; it included a 0.5-mm-thick green enveloping layer underlying the white margin, under which there was a 0.5-mm-thick yellow layer, with the deepest being an inner red layer. The concept of the layered, 3D-color-printed tooth design was to designate the cavity preparation with colored limit zones; as such, preparation of the cavity within the green zone was to be considered good preparation, preparation of the cavity within the yellow zone incomplete but not a failure, and preparation that exposes the red layer—representing the pulp chamber and pulp horns—as a clinical failure. These demarcations do not exist in conventional analog plastic teeth.

The teeth were printed using an OBJET J750 printer (Stratasys Ltd., Eden Prairie, MN, USA) utilizing Polyjet™ jetting technology, which prints models in multicolored layers with a resolution of 17 microns. The models were printed with Vero photopolymer material, creating custom-made RGB using: Black (OBJ-03286), Cyan VIVID (OBJ-03296), Magenta VIVID (OBJ-03299), Yellow VIVID (OBJ-03302), Pure White (OBJ-03327), and Support 706 (OBJ-03326) (Stratasys Ltd., Eden Prairie, MN, USA). These materials offer the following mechanical properties: modulus of elasticity = 2000–3000 MPa; flexural strength = 75–110 MPa; and tensile strength = 60–70 MPa.

2.3. Design and Method

The study evaluated the preparations of 37 dental students performing Class I amalgam cavity preparation on the mandibular left first molar as part of a complete dentition oriented in a dental mannequin head (Columbia, Dentalez, Malvern, PA, USA model AH-1-BP).

All participants performed three Class I amalgam cavity preparations on multicolored 3D-printed teeth, after undergoing a half-hour didactic lecture regarding the concept of doing so using the unique, 3D-printed, multicolored oriented teeth. Twelve participants were also randomly selected to perform the same task on two conventional plastic teeth. All preparations were performed using a micromotor handpiece (NSK, Tokyo, Japan) and straight fissure bur (330 bur, Strauss, Palm coast, FL, USA) according to the accepted preparation parameters. Participants were seated during the procedure and made use of a unit light source to simulate the actual clinical environment.

All cavity preparations were evaluated blind by two independent examiners using an explorer hand instrument without magnification; they were provided a checklist with specific criteria to result in standardized data for analysis (Appendix A). Both instructors are instructors in the operative course at the phantom laboratory. Examiners 1 and 2 have 7 and 3 years of experience as clinical instructors, respectively, although both were 10 years post-graduation.

Each preparation was initially evaluated using the prescribed checklist by each examiner; this procedure was performed a second time after 3 months under identical conditions. Examiners were blinded as to participant identity at all times.

Performance evaluation was regimented using analytical evaluation methods (checklist and criteria). The criteria examined were: outlines of cavity preparation, proportion of cavity walls, cavity depth, line angles of the cavity, directionality of the gingival floor and axial walls, injury to adjacent tooth, and finish (Appendix A). Grades were on a continuous scale of 0–100, where the passing grade was 60. Measured success of tasks was judged by depth of cavity (0.2 mm inside the dentine–enamel junction, or 1.5 mm as measured from the depth of the central groove), a marginal configuration of 90°, maintaining as much unprepared tooth structure as possible (preserving cusps and the marginal ridge), having pulpal and gingival walls perpendicular to occlusal planes, and maintaining round internal preparation angles.

2.4. Statistics

Assumptions of normality of dependent variables (students' grades) were assessed using the Kolmogorov–Smirnov test, and via visual inspections of histograms with a normal curve.

In order to assess the intra- and inter-reliability of the two examiners, an intraclass correlation coefficient (ICC) test was used [20,21].

A two-way ANOVA was used to estimate the differences in grades with the independent variables—examiners (Examiner 1, Examiner 2), and type of training model (multicolored 3D-printed teeth and regular plastic teeth)—at the first and second evaluation times.

All analyses were performed using SPSS version 20 (IBM Corp, Armonk, NY, USA). Significant differences were considered as $p < 0.05$.

3. Results

A Kolmogorov–Smirnov test performed on students' grades indicated a normal distribution ($p > 0.05$). Table 1 shows the mean, standard deviation (SD), range, and percentiles (P25, P50, and P75) of the cavity preparations' grades on multicolored 3D-printed teeth and on conventional plastic teeth by the two examiners, at the first and second evaluations.

Table 1. Mean, SD, range, and percentiles (P25, P50, and P75) of the preparations on multicolored 3D-printed teeth (N = 111) and preparations on conventional plastic teeth (N = 24) by two instructors, at the first and second evaluation times.

		First Evaluation				Second Evaluation			
		Mean (±SD) (Range)	**P25**	**P50**	**P75**	**Mean (±SD) (Range)**	**P25**	**P50**	**P75**
multicolored 3D-printed teeth (N = 111)	Examiner 1	51.6 (±23.6) (12.5–97)	30	55	72.5	44.8 (±22.4) (8.75–98)	25	41.2	63.7
	Examiner 2	47.5 (±24.4) (5–93.7)	26.2	46.2	67.5	32.7 (±18.2) (8.75–75)	18.7	27.5	45
Conventional plastic teeth (N = 24)	Examiner 1	49.7 (±28.7) (4–95)	23.7	51.8	71.8	45.4 (±21.9) (20–93)	30	36.8	65.2
	Examiner 2	31.6 (±15.9) (8–73)	20	30	35	27 (±16.2) (6–68)	14	26.2	32.1

3.1. Intra-Examiner Reliability

The intraclass correlation coefficient (ICC) is a measure (between 0 and 1) of the reliability of data to be collected as a group; the higher the value, the higher the reliability. A confidence interval (CI) of 95% was chosen to compare the means of the group's data.

The ICC for the intra-examiner reliability of Examiner 1 was significant and good on multicolored 3D-printed teeth preparations (0.716, $p = 0.0005$, 95% CI (0.61, 0.79)) and moderate on conventional plastic teeth preparations (0.612, $p = 0.001$, 95% CI (0.28, 0.89)). For examiner 2 it was significant and moderate on multicolored 3D-printed teeth preparations (0.481, $p = 0.0005$, 95% CI (0.32, 0.61)) and not significant and low on conventional plastic teeth (0.095, $p = 0.326$, 95%CI (−0.31, 0.47)).

3.2. Inter-Examiner Reliability

The ICC for inter-examiner reliability was significant and excellent between examiners for multicolored 3D-printed teeth preparations at the first (0.929, $p = 0.0005$, 95% CI (0.89, 0.95)) and second (0.768, $p = 0.0005$, 95% CI (0.67, 0.83)) evaluation times (Figure 2). For conventional plastic teeth it was not significant and low for the first evaluation (0.314 $p = 0.063$, 95% CI (−0.94, 0.63)) and significant and moderate for the second evaluation (0.672 $p = 0.0005$, 95% CI (0.376, 0.843)).

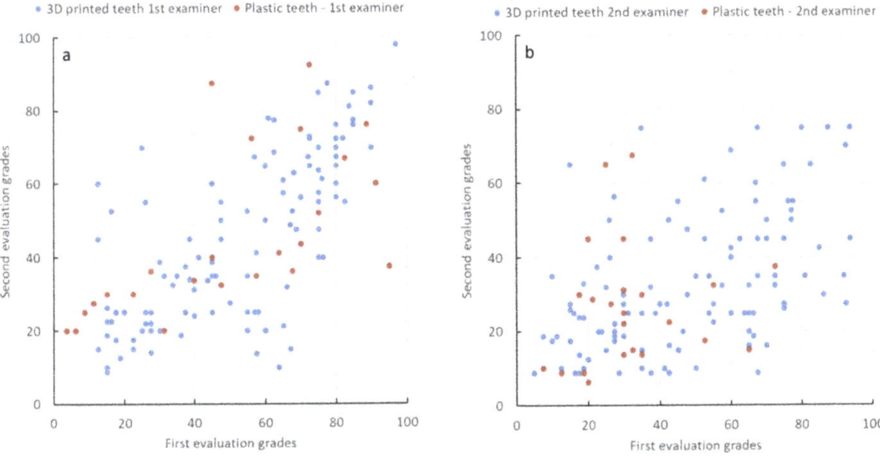

Figure 2. First vs. second preparation evaluation grades: (**a**) first examiner; (**b**) second examiner.

3.3. Effect of Examiners and Type of Training Model

A two-way ANOVA examined the effects of the examiners and the type of training model on students' grades in each evaluation time.

At the first evaluation, there was no significant interaction between the effects of the examiners and the type of training on the grades ($p = 0.066$). Simple main effects analysis showed that Examiner 1's grades were statistically significantly higher than Examiner 2's grades ($p = 0.004$), and the grades on multicolored 3D-printed teeth were statistically significantly higher than the grades on conventional plastic teeth ($p = 0.019$).

At the second evaluation, there was no significant interaction between the effects of the examiners and the type of training on the grades ($p = 0.323$). Simple main effects analysis showed that Examiner 1's grades were statistically significantly higher than Examiner 2's grades ($p = 0.0005$), but there were no differences between the type of training on grades ($p = 0.428$).

4. Discussion

The purpose of preclinical dental courses is to simulate as closely as possible the actual circumstances that patient care entails. The use of mannequins as representative of human head anatomy is the classic method of presenting dental students with these parameters. Included in this model are replicas of the jaws and teeth, on which instruction is given by skilled educators as to the steps required to perform appropriate dental preparations [6].

The most common mode of this type of education is to observe the instructor as they perform and explain the needed tasks. Furthermore, said instructors are required to evaluate each student's endeavors in order to gauge their progress. However, the majority of instructors are solo practitioners, which tends to produce uneven standards in technique and insular scales of evaluation. Previous studies have described the educational shortcomings of evaluating preclinical dental student performance due to inconsistency within and among examiners [9–11]. In addition, the use of magnifications (i.e., loupes) for evaluating cavity preparation might further enhance the procedure [22].

The present study is an effort to alleviate the issues of the reliability and accuracy of the evaluation of clinical performance by instructors. The former refers to the consistency of earned marks regardless of who administers them or when [20]. To fulfill this definition, we developed a novel analog model of human teeth with multicolored layers using 3D digital printing. These are designed to follow the margins of an ideal cavity preparation (border of white and green) in all dimensions, with strata of green, yellow, and red beneath an outer ivory surface [19]. The removal of material from these analogs provides both student and instructor with direct visual feedback as to the performance of the given procedure. The ability to discern even minor deviations in this manner is superior to and more objective than the traditional method using monochromatic plastic teeth.

The results of this study show that, by using the novel multicolored 3D-printed teeth, both intra- and inter-examiner reliability was improved. Cicchetti (1994) [23] described commonly cited ranges for the qualitative rating of agreement based on ICC values, i.e., "good" for values between 0.6 and 0.74, and "excellent" for values between 0.75 and 1. In our study, the ICC was used to measure the inter-examiner reliability in both the multicolored 3D-printed and the conventional plastic teeth. The agreement between examiners was found to be excellent for both the first (ICC = 0.929), and second (ICC = 0.768) evaluations on multicolored 3D-printed teeth. When conventional plastic teeth were used to test this, it was found to be low at the first (ICC = 0.314) and moderate at the second (ICC = 0.672) evaluations.

These findings are different from those reported by Lee et al. (2018) [21], who reported that inter-examiner reliability was excellent for both methods of digital assessment by CEREC software and conventional visual assessment of cavity preparation on regular plastic teeth (ICC from 0.77–0.87). However, Zou et al. (2016) [24], who compared a conventional visual assessment with a computerized laser-scanning cavity preparation skill evaluation system (CPSES) of class I cavity preparation by clinical instructors, reported that the CPSES gave consistent inter-examiner reliability and excellent intra-examiner reliability (ICC 1), in contrast to the conventional method (ICC from 0.56 to 0.77).

The use of digital tools in modern dentistry permits the rapid scanning of student cavity preparation and comparison with standardized cavity preparation models. This can generate 3D feedback data using computer-based evaluation systems such as PrepCheck [15], CEREC [21], and CPSES [24]. Previous studies have indicated that this method provides more consistent and accurate grading [25,26]; however, they require significant training before usage, standardization of variation among independent instructors now needing to alter individual variability in teaching habits, increased time needed to obtain digital feedback and high costs. Consequently, digital assessment should not replace conventional methods; rather, it can overlap these as a supplemental method of evaluation.

The aim of developing the novel, multicolored 3D-printed teeth was to replace the conventional monochromatic plastic teeth in order to facilitate a more objective and accurate evaluation method, while still using the traditional assessment method by both students and instructors. Moreover, the conventional assessment method more closely follows actual clinical practice. Hence, the novel multicolored 3D-printed tooth analogs enable assessment in the same manner as with conventional plastic teeth, while providing more objective and accurate evaluation of cavity preparation.

Intra-examiner reliability is determined by comparing the grades given by an examiner of the same object at one point in time with those given at another significantly separated point in time. In the present study, this was done 3 months apart. Furthermore, the examiners who participated in the present study were of different levels of expertise (Examiner 1 was considered to have more expertise), because previous studies have reported that experience improved intra-examiner reliability, and less experienced examiners have been shown to be more inconsistent [20]. Our findings are consistent with those previously reported, as Examiner 1 displayed more intra-examiner reliability (ICC = 0.716 on multicolored teeth and 0.612 on regular teeth) than Examiner 2 (ICC = 0.481 on multicolored teeth and 0.095 on regular teeth).

Our findings suggest that examiner/instructor influence is the main factor correlated to the grades given to dental student cavity preparations. Furthermore, it was found that the novel, multicolored 3D-printed tooth analogs increase the level of consistency of the less experienced examiner. The explanation for the improvement by the less experienced examiner with the 3D model is that it provides an alternative means to assess student performance over the conventional method of assessment. The multicolored 3D-printed teeth provided additional visual feedback on performance success and errors according to the various color layers exposed inside the cavity. These make the dimensions, depth, and location of the tooth preparation more clear for both student and teacher, thus facilitating more objective and accurate evaluation of tooth preparation.

5. Conclusions

1. The novel, multicolored 3D-printed tooth analogs can provide a more objective evaluation of cavity preparation compared with conventional plastic teeth. The novel, multicolored 3D-printed teeth could improve the current evaluation method for assessing undergraduate skills by improving examiner consistency.
2. Although intra-examiner unreliability persists, the use of this novel, multicolored 3D-printed tooth analog might reduce it, especially with less experienced instructors.

Author Contributions: Conceptualization, D.L. and T.B.; methodology, D.L., T.B. and R.P.; investigation, M.A.; data curation, D.L., A.S. and M.A.; writing—original draft preparation, M.A., D.L. and T.B.; writing—review and editing, D.L., R.P., A.S., M.D. and T.B.; visualization, M.D.; supervision, T.B. and R.P.; project administration, D.L. and A.S.; funding acquisition, T.B. and R.P. All authors have read and agreed to the published version of the manuscript.

Funding: This study was partially supported by a grant provided by the Ministry of Science, Technology and Space, Israel, Grant number: 3-12439.

Institutional Review Board Statement: The study was conducted according to the guidelines and approved by the Institutional Ethics Committee of Tel Aviv University (12 February 2018).

Informed Consent Statement: Informed consent was obtained from all subjects involved in the study.

Data Availability Statement: Data available on request due to restrictions eg privacy or ethical. The data presented in this study are available on request from the corresponding author. The data are not publicly available due to privacy of the students' grades.

Acknowledgments: This study was partially supported by a grant provided by the Ministry of Science, Technology, and Space, Israel, grant number: 3-12439. The authors would like to acknowledge the contributions of the engineer Yosi Kamir, from the School of Chemistry, and the industrial designer Raz Silberman, from SYNERGY studio, for planning the 3D-printed tooth models for the research.

Conflicts of Interest: The authors declare no conflict of interest.

Appendix A. Class I—Cavity Feedback Form

Number of preparation:
Student number:

Outline	A	B	C	D
All the caries and the continuous cracks have been removed				
There is no redundant tooth material				
Round edges				
Cavity Walls				
Compatible with the tooth length axis				
Correct diversion				
Smoothness				
Cavity Floor				
Depth				
Smoothness				
Round line angles				

References

1. Spratley, M.H. Aptitude testing and the selection of dental students. *Aust. Dent. J.* **1990**, *35*, 159–168. [CrossRef]
2. Boyle, A.M.; Santelli, J.C. Assessing psychomotor skills: The role of the Crawford small parts dexterity test as a screening instruments. *J. Dent. Educ.* **1985**, *50*, 176–179. [CrossRef]
3. Schwibbe, A.; Kothe, C.; Hampe, W.; Konradt, U. Acquisition of dental skills in preclinical technique courses: Influence of spatial and manual abilities. *Adv. Health Sci. Educ. Theory Pract.* **2016**, *21*, 841–857. [CrossRef]
4. Suddick, R.P.; Yancey, J.M.; Wilson, S. Mirror tracing and embedded figures tests as predictors of dental students' performance. *J. Dent. Educ.* **1983**, *47*, 149–154. [CrossRef] [PubMed]
5. Peterson, S. The ADA chalk carving test. *J. Dent. Educ.* **1974**, *38*, 11–15. [CrossRef]
6. Suvinen, T.I.; Messer, L.B.; Franco, E. Clinical simulation in teaching preclinical dentistry. *Eur. J. Dent. Educ.* **1998**, *2*, 25–32. [CrossRef]
7. Mocny-Pachońska, K.; Doniec, R.; Trzcionka, A.; Pachoński, M.; Piaseczna, N.; Sieciński, S.; Osadcha, O.; Łanowy, P.; Tanasiewicz, M. Evaluating the stress-response of dental students to the dental school environment. *PeerJ* **2020**, *8*, e8981. [CrossRef]
8. Mocny-Pacho´nska, K.; Doniec, R.J.; Wójcik, S.; Sieci´nski, S.; Piaseczna, N.J.; Duraj, K.M.; Tkacz, E.J. Evaluation of the most stressful dental treatment procedures of conservative dentistry among Polish dental students. *Int. J. Environ. Res. Public Health* **2021**, *18*, 4448. [CrossRef] [PubMed]
9. Sharaf, A.A.; Abdelaziz, A.M.; El Meligy, O.A.S. Intra- and inter-examiner variability in evaluating preclinical pediatric dentistry operative procedures. *J. Dent. Educ.* **2007**, *71*, 540–544. [CrossRef]
10. Jenkins, S.M.; Dummer, P.M.H.; Gilmour, A.S.M.; Edmunds, D.H.; Hicks, R.; Ash, P. Evaluating undergraduate preclinical operative skill; use of a glance and grade marking system. *J. Dent.* **1996**, *26*, 679–684. [CrossRef]
11. Vann, W.F.; Machen, J.B.; Hounshell, P.B. Effects of criteria and checklists on reliability in preclinical evaluation. *J. Dent. Educ.* **1983**, *47*, 671–675. [CrossRef] [PubMed]

12. Salvendy, G.; Hinton, W.M.; Ferguson, G.W.; Cunningham, P.R. Pilot study on criteria in cavity preparation–Facts or artifacts? *J. Dent. Educ.* **1973**, *37*, 27–31. [CrossRef]
13. Cervino, G.; Fiorillo, L.; Arzukanyan, A.V.; Spagnuolo, G.; Cicciù, M. Dental restorative digital workflow: Digital smile design from aesthetic to function. *Dent. J.* **2019**, *7*, 30. [CrossRef]
14. Wolgin, M.; Frank, W.; Kielbassa, A.M. Development of an analytical prepCheck-supported approach to evaluate tutor-based assessments of dental students' practical skills. *Int. J. Comput. Dent.* **2018**, *21*, 313–322. [PubMed]
15. Cardoso, J.A.; Barbosa, C.; Fernandes, S.; Silva, C.L.; Pinho, A. Reducing subjectivity in the evaluation of pre-clinical dental preparations for fixed prosthodontics using the Kavo PrepAssistant. *Eur. J. Dent. Educ.* **2006**, *10*, 149–156. [CrossRef] [PubMed]
16. Kunkel, T.C.; Engelmeier, R.L.; Shah, N.H. A comparison of crown preparation grading via prepCheck versus grading by dental school instructors. *Int. J. Comput. Dent.* **2018**, *21*, 305–311.
17. Wolgin, M.; Grabowski, S.; Elhadad, S.; Frank, W.; Kielbassa, A.M. Comparison of a prepCheck supported self-assessment concept with conventional faculty supervision in a pre-clinical simulation environment. *Eur. J. Dent. Educ.* **2018**, *22*, e522–e529. [CrossRef]
18. Lugassy, D.; Levanon, Y.; Rosen, G.; Livne, S.; Fridenberg, N.; Pilo, R.; Brosh, T. Does augmented visual feedback from novel, multicolored, three-dimensional-printed teeth affect dental students' acquisition of manual skills? *Anat. Sci. Educ.* **2020**, *31*. online ahead of print. [CrossRef]
19. Singh, P.; Sehgal, G.V. Black caries classification and preparation technique using optimal CNN-LSTM classifier. *Multimed. Tools Appl.* **2021**, *80*, 5255–5272. [CrossRef]
20. Taylor, C.L.; Grey, N.; Satterthwaite, J.D. Assessing the clinical skills of dental students: A review of the literature. *J. Educ. Learn.* **2013**, *2*, 20–31. [CrossRef]
21. Lee, C.; Kobayashi, H.; Lee, S.R.; Ohyama, H. The role of digital 3D scanned models in dental students' self-assessments in preclinical operative dentistry. *J. Dent. Educ.* **2018**, *82*, 399–405. [CrossRef] [PubMed]
22. Cicchetti, D.V. Guidelines, criteria and rules of thumb for evaluating normed and standardized assessment instruments in psychology. *Psych. Assess.* **1994**, *6*, 284–290. [CrossRef]
23. Lo Giudice, G.; Lo Giudice, R.; Matarese, G.; Isola, G.; Cicciù, M.; Terranova, A.; Palaia, G.; Romeo, U. Evaluation of magnification systems in restorative dentistry. An in-vitro study. *Dental. Cadmos.* **2015**, *83*, 296–305. [CrossRef]
24. Zou, H.; Jin, S.; Sun, J.; Dai, Y. A cavity preparation evaluation system in the skill assessment of dental students. *J. Dent. Educ.* **2016**, *80*, 930–937. [CrossRef]
25. Hamil, L.M.; Mennito, A.S.; Renne, W.G.; Jompobe, V. Dental students' opinions of preparation assessment with E4D compare software versus traditional methods. *J. Dent. Educ.* **2014**, *78*, 1424–1431. [CrossRef]
26. Mays, K.A.; Levine, E. Dental students' self-assessment of operative preparations using CAD/CAM: A preliminary analysis. *J. Dent. Educ.* **2014**, *78*, 1673–1680. [CrossRef] [PubMed]

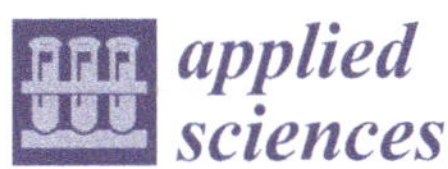

applied sciences

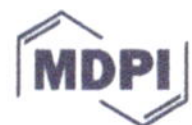

Article

A Proposed In Vitro Methodology for Assessing the Accuracy of Three-Dimensionally Printed Dental Models and the Impact of Storage on Dimensional Stability

Li Hsin Lin [1], Joshua Granatelli [1], Frank Alifui-Segbaya [1], Laura Drake [2], Derek Smith [2] and Khaled E. Ahmed [1,*]

[1]   School of Medicine and Dentistry, Griffith University, Gold Coast, QLD 4215, Australia;
      leo.lin@griffithuni.edu.au (L.H.L.); joshua.granatelli@griffithuni.edu.au (J.G.);
      f.alifui-segbaya@griffith.edu.au (F.A.-S.)
[2]   Advanced Design and Prototyping Technologies Institute, Griffith University,
      Gold Coast, QLD 4215, Australia; l.drake@griffith.edu.au (L.D.); derek.smith@griffith.edu.au (D.S.)
*   Correspondence: khaled.ahmed@griffith.edu.au; Tel.: +61-7-5678-0596

Abstract: The objective of this study was to propose a standardised methodology for assessing the accuracy of three-dimensional printed (3DP) full-arch dental models and the impact of storage using two printing technologies. A reference model (RM) comprising seven spheres was 3D-printed using digital light processing (MAX UV, MAX) and stereolithography (Form 2, F2) five times per printer. The diameter of the spheres ($n = 35$) represented the dimensional trueness (DT), while twenty-one vectors ($n = 105$) extending between the sphere centres represented the full-arch trueness (FT). Samples were measured at two (T_1) and six (T_2) weeks using a commercial profilometer to assess their dimensional stability. Significant ($p < 0.05$) contraction in DT occurred at T_1 and T_2 with a medium deviation of 108 μm and 99 μm for MAX, and 117 μm and 118 μm for F2, respectively. No significant ($p > 0.05$) deviations were detected for FT. The detected median deviations were evenly distributed across the arch for MAX at <50 μm versus F2, where the greatest error of 278 μm was in the posterior region. Storage did not significantly impact the model's DT in contrast to FT ($p < 0.05$). The proposed methodology was able to assess the accuracy of 3DP. Storage significantly impacted the full-arch accuracy of the models up to 6 weeks post-printing.

Keywords: three-dimensional printing; dimensional stability; dental models; methodology; accuracy; storage

Citation: Lin, L.H.; Granatelli, J.; Alifui-Segbaya, F.; Drake, L.; Smith, D.; Ahmed, K.E. A Proposed In Vitro Methodology for Assessing the Accuracy of Three-Dimensionally Printed Dental Models and the Impact of Storage on Dimensional Stability. *Appl. Sci.* **2021**, *11*, 5994. https://doi.org/10.3390/app11135994

Academic Editor: Kathrin Becker

Received: 30 May 2021
Accepted: 25 June 2021
Published: 28 June 2021

Publisher's Note: MDPI stays neutral with regard to jurisdictional claims in published maps and institutional affiliations.

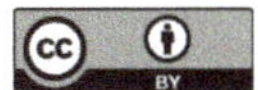

1. Introduction

Whether fully digital or hybrid, the digital workflow offers a valuable opportunity for cost-effective and streamlined delivery of dental care. Three-dimensional printing (3DP) is part of the digital workflow, which is being adopted into the dental industry at a rapid rate [1]. 3DP is an additive process involving layer-by-layer (z-axis) deposition of material in the x- and y-axes [2,3]. The fabrication of 3D printed dental models for single crowns, fixed and removable partial dentures, surgical guides, orthodontic aligners, and treatment planning are examples of the adoption of this technology in routine practise [4,5].

Multiple printing technologies have been developed for 3DP, with one of the most established to date being photopolymerisation [6]. Stereolithography (SLA) and digital light processing (DLP) are common photopolymerisation-based 3DP systems [3,7,8]. SLA involves galvanometer mirrors that direct ultraviolet light to selectively polymerise the monomers point by point across the x-y axis before the build platform moves into the z-axis to incrementally build the appliance [1,9]. In contrast, DLP utilises micromirrors to direct the projector light to polymerise the entire x-y layer all at once, resulting in a reduced production time compared to SLA [1,10].

The accuracy of 3D printed dental models has been extensively researched, with a recent systematic review identifying their accuracy varies significantly, between <100 and

>500 μm, not only between different printing technologies but also within studies evaluating similar 3D printers [1]. Etemad-Shahidi et al. [1] attributed this to the heterogeneity of the study designs in the included studies, which led to a high risk of bias, calling for standardised testing and reporting protocol in studies investigating 3DP accuracy.

Furthermore, there is currently limited evidence in the existing literature investigating the impact of storage on the dimensional stability of 3D printed dental models [1,11]. Additionally, and to the authors' knowledge, no studies have investigated the full-arch dimensional stability of 3D printed models. As stated by Joda et al. [11], the fabrication of all types of dental prostheses and appliances is currently not plausible solely through the digital workflow, often requiring analogue input. Therefore, in cases where a combination of analogue and digital workflow is required, the dimensional stability of 3D printed models becomes of direct clinical interest. The dimensional stability of 3D printed models is of critical importance in cases of limited access to 3D printers where service delays are inevitable: increased workload, lack of in-house facilities, and shipping needs of rural and outreach locations. Further complicating the streamlining of the hybrid workflow is the potentially extended time needed for the actual printing of the dental model, inherently dependant on the printing system available, and could span to several hours per model. Henceforth, it is paramount that a 3D printed model remains dimensionally stable during storage to ensure the proper fabrication of the prosthesis for adequate seating, conformity with the patient's stomatognathic system and the planned treatment especially in multi-unit indirect restoration that requires a passive fit upon insertion, and surgical guides for accurate implant placement [11,12]. If, however, 3D printed models do demonstrate dimensional changes with storage, then such changes should be accounted for as part of the validation process of the workflow.

The objective of this study was to propose a standardised methodology for assessing the accuracy of 3D printed full-arch dental models and the impact of storage on the dimensional stability using two commercially available 3D printing systems.

2. Materials and Methods

2.1. Reference Model

The reference model was based on a previously published protocol [13] in the form of a horseshoe-shaped model that fits in a standard, medium-sized dental impression stock tray to mimic the dimensions of the dental arch. The STL file of the model was designed using Solidworks (Dassault Systeme, Velizy Villacoublay, France) comprising of a 6.5 mm thick base and seven spheres, approximately 10 mm in diameter, embedded in the base and distributed across the arch to represent the anterior and posterior region of the dentition (Figure 1). The diameter of each sphere, along with the vectors that extend between the hypothetical centres of the spheres of the STL file, were confirmed using surface-matching software (Geomagic Control X, 2014; 3D Systems, Rock Hill, SC, USA) (Tables 1 and 2).

Table 1. Reference measurements for the diameter of each sphere based on the reference model.

Sphere	Diameter (mm)
S_1	9.976
S_2	9.985
S_3	9.956
S_4	9.977
S_5	9.959
S_6	9.982
S_7	9.967

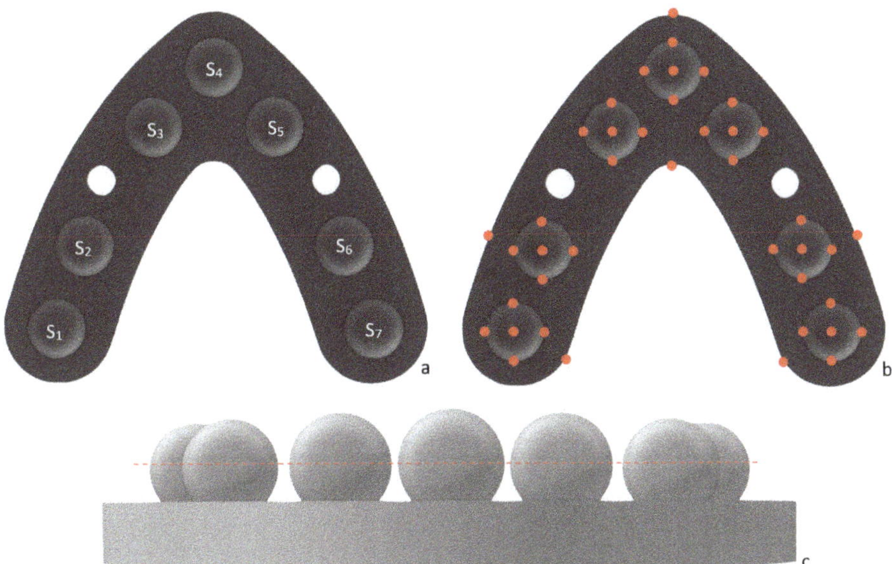

Figure 1. STL image of the reference model. (**a**) Labelled spheres where S_1, S_2, S_6 and S_7 represent the posterior region of the model while S_3–S_5 represent the anterior region. Attachment vents are present between S_2–S_3 and S_5–S_6. (**b**) Red markings indicating the location for the coordinate measuring machine measurements. (**c**) Dotted red line indicating the equator of the spheres.

Table 2. Definition of the 21 vectors extending between the hypothetical spheres centre and the corresponding reference measurements based on the reference model.

Vector	Name	Measurement (mm)
S_1–S_2	V_1	14.856
S_1–S_3	V_2	38.022
S_1–S_4	V_3	51.889
S_1–S_5	V_4	51.003
S_1–S_6	V_5	51.914
S_1–S_7	V_6	55.003
S_2–S_3	V_7	23.344
S_2–S_4	V_8	37.513
S_2–S_5	V_9	38.610
S_2–S_6	V_{10}	44.999
S_2–S_7	V_{11}	51.929
S_3–S_4	V_{12}	14.493
S_3–S_5	V_{13}	21.002
S_3–S_6	V_{14}	38.583
S_3–S_7	V_{15}	50.990
S_4–S_5	V_{16}	14.500
S_4–S_6	V_{17}	37.502
S_4–S_7	V_{18}	51.887
S_5–S_6	V_{19}	23.330
S_5–S_7	V_{20}	38.016
S_6–S_7	V_{21}	14.860

2.2. Manufacturing 3D Printed Full-Arch Dental Models

Two 3D printers utilising different 3D technologies were assessed: Form 2 (405 nm violet laser, 140 μm laser spot size; Formlabs, Somerville, MA, USA) and MAX UV (385 nm ultraviolet laser; Asiga, Alexandria, New South Wales, Australia) with SLA and DLP systems, respectively, were selected. The STL file of the reference model was imported into Form 2 slicing software (PreForm, Formlabs, Somerville, MA, USA) and the Asiga MAX UV slicing software (Asgia Composer, Asiga, Alexandria, New South Wales, Australia). The slicing software were used to orientate the model at 0 degrees/horizontally with the model base directly on the build platform. The z-axis resolution was set and standardised at 50 μm. Formlabs dental model resin (Formlabs, Sommerville, MA, USA) was used for Form 2 and Fotodent model 385/405 nm resin (Dreve, Unna, Germany) for MAX UV.

The printed models remained in the printer to drip for at least 10 min as recommended by the manufacturer to reduce resin remnant on the models. All models were then washed manually in two baths of 99.5% isopropanol (Thermo Fisher Scientific Australia, Victoria, Australia). MAX UV models were washed for 6 min (total = 12 min) and Form 2 models for 10 min (total = 20 min) in each bath. The MAX UV models were air-dried before post-curing for 10 min with a light-curing unit (Otoflash G171, 280–700 nm, Puretone 3D, Kent, United Kingdom) under nitrogen gas with a total of 6000 flashes. The Form 2 models were post-cured in LC-3D Print Box (NextDent, 315–550 nm, Soesterberg, The Netherlands) for 10 min.

2.3. Assessment of Accuracy

Each sample model comprised 7 spheres and 21 vector measurements extending between the hypothetical sphere centres. Five models ($n = 5$) were printed for each printer to assess the dimensional ($n = 35$) and full-arch accuracy ($n = 105$). The printed models were measured using a coordinate measuring machine (CMM, Absolute Arm 7-Axis, Hexagon, Cobham, UK) with a 50 mm long probe and a 3 mm ruby tip within two weeks (T_1) of printing. The Absolute Arm 7-Axis was calibrated according to ISO 10360-12 with a confirmed error of 0.005 mm. The CMM measurements began by outlining the base of the model to establish an area in space on PolyWorks Inspector (Innovmetric, QC, Canada) using six points circumferentially around the base of the model. The dimensions of the spheres were then measured using nine points with four points circumferentially below the equator, four points circumferentially above the equator, and one point at the top-centre of the sphere (Figure 1). The sequence of measurements was from S_1 through to S_7. The S_1 location was then combined with the line vector from S_1 to S_7 to create a cartesian axis located in the measured centre of S_1. The diameter of the spheres was then calculated using the sphere function on PolyWorks Inspector. The hypothetical centre of each sphere was then used to measure the 21 vectors listed in Table 2 on PolyWorks. All models were stored and measured in a temperature-controlled room (24 °C, 1013 hPa), with the same operator completing all measurements. The 3D printed models were stored in the same conditions in a dark storage compartment devoid of light, then measured again six weeks (T_2) after printing to assess the dimensional stability of 3D printed models.

The diameter of the spheres was used to assess the dimensional accuracy of the printed models. The full-arch accuracy was assessed based on the combination of the 21 vectors that extended between the hypothetical sphere centres. Specific arch segments were also assessed to identify the pattern of changes through a combination of different cross-arch vectors: left posterior (V_1, V_2, V_7), right posterior (V_{19}, V_{20}, V_{21}), posterior (V_5, V_6, V_{10}, V_{11}), anterior (V_{12}, V_{13}, V_{16}), and anteroposterior (V_3, V_{18}).

2.4. Statistical Analysis

The median deviation was used to assess the trueness, and the interquartile range (IQR) was used to determine the precision. The normality of the data was evaluated using the Shapiro–Wilk test. One-sample Wilcoxon signed-rank test was used to compare the dimensional and full-arch trueness of the two printing systems at T_1 and T_2 against the reference measurements. The dimensional and full-arch accuracy of the two printing systems were compared using the Mann–Whitney U test. The same test was used to assess significant differences between the left and right posterior arch segments and anterior and posterior arch segments. The dimensional stability of the 3D printed model between T_1 and T_2 was assessed using Wilcoxon signed-rank test. All statistical analysis was performed using IBM SPSS statistics software (Version 24; IBM, Armonk, NY, USA) with a significance level of 0.05.

3. Results

The dimensional trueness of both tested printing systems was statistically different from the reference measurement ($p < 0.05$) at both time points. MAX UV demonstrated median deviation of 108 μm and 99 μm whilst Form 2 yielded 117 μm and 118 μm at two- and six-weeks post-printing, respectively. The study found no significant difference from the reference model ($p > 0.05$) for either 3D printer at both two- and six-weeks post-printing in terms of full-arch trueness.

Comparison of the dimensional accuracy between the two printing systems resulted in a statistical difference ($p = 0.005$). MAX UV had a lower median deviation (108 μm) and greater precision (27 μm) when compared to Form 2, which had trueness of 117 μm and precision of 59 μm after two weeks post-printing (Figure 2). Similarly, a statistical difference ($p = 0.000$) was also present for full-arch accuracy, with MAX UV having a smaller error (26 μm) and higher precision (32 μm) (Figure 3).

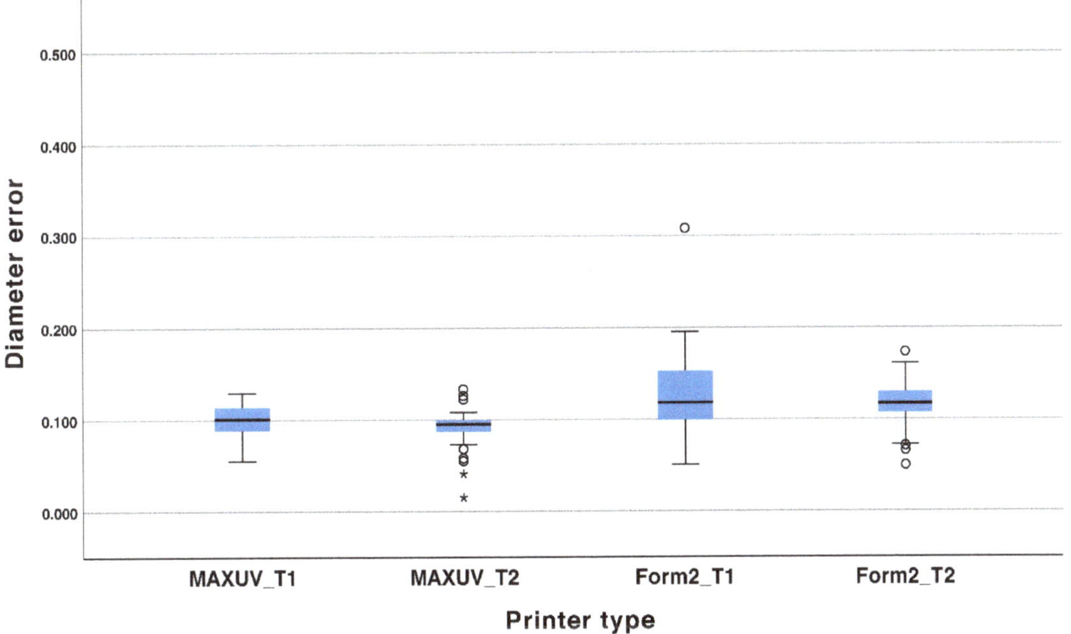

Figure 2. Boxplot for the median error and precision of the sphere diameter at T1 and T2 for MAX UV and Form 2 3D printed models. ° Denotes outliers more than 1.5 IQR but less than three IQR from the end of the boxplot. * Denotes outliers more than three IQR from the end of the boxplot.

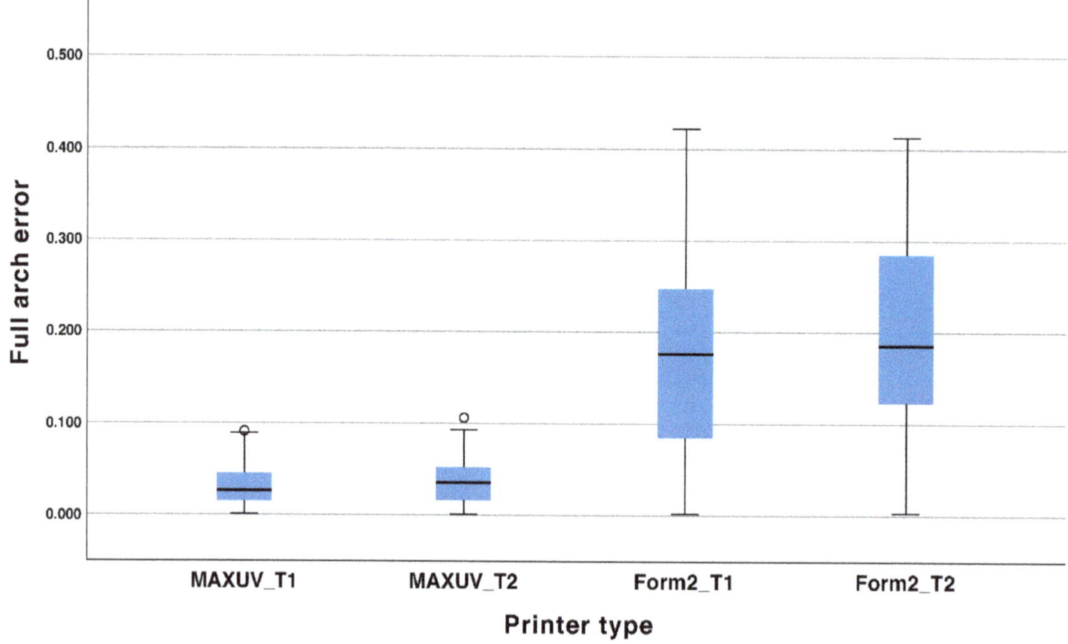

Figure 3. Boxplot for the median error and precision of the full-arch parameter at T_1 (two weeks post-printing) and T_2 (six weeks post-printing) for MAX UV and Form 2 3D printed models. ° Denotes outliers more than 1.5 IQR but less than three IQR from the end of the boxplot.

When the models were stored for an additional four weeks after the initial measurement, no statistical differences were found for the dimensional deviation between the two time points for both printers ($p > 0.05$). However, statistical differences were detected for full-arch accuracy for both MAX UV samples ($p = 0.003$) and Form 2 samples ($p = 0.000$) between two- and six-weeks post-printing indicating a progressive contraction with time (Figures 2 and 3).

The analysis of the individual arch segments did not identify significant differences ($p > 0.05$) in the deviation between the left and right posterior arch for both printers. Similarly, no statistical difference ($p = 0.117$) was found between the anterior and posterior arch for MAX UV. However, Form 2 showed significant ($p = 0.000$) posterior cross-arch shrinkage when the anterior (vectors V_{12}, V_{13}, V_{16}) and posterior arch (vectors V_5, V_6, V_{10}, V_{11}) segments were compared (Table 3). The Form 2 models also showed a large anteroposterior (vector V_3, V_{18}) contraction with a median deviation of 212 µm from the reference measurement with low precision of 124 µm.

Table 3. Median deviation and interquartile range (IQR) of arch segments: left posterior; right posterior; posterior; anterior; anteroposterior of MAX UV and Form 2 3D printed models at T_1.

Printer	Measurements	Left Posterior	Right Posterior	Posterior	Anterior	Anteroposterior
Max UV	Median deviation (µm)	20	9	49	27	23
	IQR (µm)	31	12	47	27	31
	p-value		0.152		0.117	
Form 2	Median deviation (µm)	94	114	278	56	212
	IQR (µm)	76	157	94	88	124
	p-value		0.576		0.000	

The tested DLP system was more than twice as efficient as the SLA system with similar resin consumptions. MAX UV required approximately 37.7 mL of resin for the fabrication of two models in 1 h and 48 min. On the other hand, Form 2 required 37.3 mL to fabricate two models in 4 h.

4. Discussion

The aim of this study was to propose a standardised testing methodology for assessing the accuracy of 3D printed full-arch dental models and the impact of storage on them. The current study utilised the combination of metrology and 3D linear measurements using an industrial coordinate measuring machine and inspection software as a gold standard to reduce the error associated with physical calliper measurements and best-fit superimposition [14–16]. Previous studies have relied on the best-fit (iterative closest point) algorithm for superimposition, which may compensate positive deviations and negative ones resulting in the under- or over-estimation of errors [16,17]. On the other hand, physical, digital calliper measurements have been criticised for their poor repeatability, reliance on reference areas that may change over time, and limited access to small areas on the models [18]. The use of varying typodont models in different studies presents significant challenges to the standardisation of testing and meaningful comparison among studies. Henceforth, the current study proposed the use of simple, spherical geometry that can be readily replicated to determine the highest possible accuracy of 3DP whilst avoiding the use of complex tooth morphology that may introduce a greater risk of variation and measurement error [13,19]. Indeed, the choice of spherical geometry was based on the accuracy testing methodology adopted by the International Organization for Standardization in several of its standards, which involves the measurement of spheres, including ISO12836:2015 annex C evaluating *digitizing devices for CAD/CAM systems for indirect dental restorations* and ISO10360:2009/2020 parts 2 and 5 for *acceptance and reverification tests for coordinate measuring systems (CMS)*. The methodology employed in the current study was also previously validated for assessing the dimensional accuracy and stability of Type IV stone dental models, presenting a suitable follow-up in the assessment of 3D printed dental models [13]. The proposed methodology relied on a direct comparison between the 3D printed samples and the STL image of the reference model, subsequently eliminating errors arising from the scanning of a physical reference model such as scanning system error, the dimensional stability of a stone cast, optical properties of the reference model, operator influence, or light conditions [6,13,20–24].

The dimensional trueness identified in the current study with an error of <120 μm concurred with the accuracy findings reported in similar studies [25,26]. Additionally, for full-arch accuracy, the detected anteroposterior and cross-arch dimensional contraction associated with the SLA printer was also identified in previous studies [16,27,28]. This cross-arch contraction progressively increased towards the posterior aspect as the model diverged, resulting in a reduction in cross-arch support, which was also reported by Papaspyridakos et al. [16]. However, the study by Kim et al. [25] reported greater cross-arch trueness for their SLA printer (ZENITH; Dentis, Daegu, Korea) when compared to their DLP printer (M-ONE; MAKEX Technology, Ningbo, Zhejiang, China). Therefore, the cause of the dimensional distortion for the tested Form 2 models is more likely associated with the resin formulation as the investigation from Lin et al. [29] suggested that different compositions of ethoxylated bisphenol A-dimethacrylate, triethylene glycol dimethacrylate, and urethane dimethacrylate may influence the accuracy of 3DP. Moreover, Reymus et al. [30] reported that the choice of post-curing method played a significant role in the degree of conversion of the photo-sensitive resin – with the Otoflash G171 demonstrating the greatest degree of conversion versus the LC-3D Print Box being the lowest, which possibly explained the delayed dimensional changes identified in the study. The similarities between the results of the current study and literature supports the ability of the simple spherical geometry to assess the dimensional distortion of 3D printed models.

The present study also investigated the dimensional stability of 3D printed models using two printing systems over a period of six weeks. Currently, there are limited data in the literature investigating the dimensional stability of 3D printed models. The dimensional stability of 3D printed models is a clinically important parameter. The study by Jang et al. [31] showed that, although the fit of crowns produced on 3D printed models was acceptable, it remains inferior to conventional dies. This might be attributed to the detected dimensional errors of 3DP that need to be accounted for during the fabrication process of extra-coronal restoration to achieve better fitting restoration with minimal internal and marginal discrepancies. In the current study, the diameter of the seven spheres represents the short-span accuracy, as well as the twenty-one vectors extending between the centres of the seven spheres, representing the full-arch parameter of 3DP, was investigated to elucidate the pattern of dimensional changes exhibited for SLA and DLP manufactured dental models. No significant difference was detected for the diameter of the spheres between 2 weeks and 6 weeks indicating that for short-span application, any errors arising from model storage are expected to be within the reported clinically acceptable thresholds of 120 µm [32,33] and supporting their suitability, from an accuracy perceptive, for single crown and short-span application irrespective of storage time. Furthermore, for both SLA and DLP printers, the magnitude of the detected dimensional changes was similar to those reported for type IV die stone over 8 weeks of storage [34], albeit stone models exhibited expansion, as opposed to the contraction exhibited by 3DP. In contrast, the full-arch findings indicate significant and delayed contraction for both printing systems after storage and in agreement with similar in vitro studies [11,17]. The SLA models in this study exhibited significant contraction in an anteroposterior and cross-arch direction, in contrast to DLP which contracted evenly. Such contraction may impact the fit of full-arch appliances and restorations fabricated using these 3DP models due to their localised and skewed error pattern of >200 µm. On the other hand, the dimensional stability results of the DLP printer were within the clinically acceptable error margin of 59–150 µm [16] required for accuracy-demanding prosthodontic application such as implant-retained fixed prosthesis even after six weeks of storage. These findings do support the notion that a clear understanding of the performance and limitation of the 3D printing system is cardinal for determining their most suitable dental application and the timing of the manufacturing workflow.

The main limitation of this study is its in vitro nature and the reliance on simple object geometry for a reference model. Hence, whilst the methodology facilitates reproduction and standardisation of testing, the derived results represent ideal testing conditions that do not account for other clinical factors such as complex dental morphology and the presence of orthodontic crowding. Moreover, a limitation shared with similar studies is the applicability of the results to the resins used, which, albeit recommended by the manufacturers of the tested SLA and DLP printers for full-arch models, may not fully represent the array of printing resins currently in the market. Future research should be aimed at establishing the effect of different variables such as other resins and alternative post-processing methods on the accuracy of 3D printed full-arch models.

5. Conclusions

Within the limitations of in vitro testing conditions, the proposed methodology was able to assess the accuracy of 3D printed full-arch dental models, identifying greater accuracy with the tested DLP printer. The 3D printed models demonstrated continued dimensional changes over a period of 6 weeks irrespective of the printing system used. Whilst 3DP produced highly accurate models, caution should be exercised when utilising them after prolonged storage, for long-span or full-arch prostheses and appliances, and model analyses.

Author Contributions: Conceptualisation, K.E.A.; methodology, L.H.L., J.G., F.A.-S., L.D., D.S. and K.E.A.; software, L.D. and D.S.; validation, L.H.L. and K.E.A.; formal analysis, L.H.L. and J.G.; investigation, L.H.L. and J.G.; resources, K.E.A.; data curation, L.H.L., J.G. and L.D.; writing—original draft preparation, L.H.L.; writing—review and editing, L.H.L., J.G., F.A.-S., L.D., D.S. and K.E.A.; visualisation, L.H.L. and J.G.; supervision, F.A.-S. and K.E.A.; project administration, K.E.A.; funding acquisition, K.E.A. All authors have read and agreed to the published version of the manuscript.

Funding: This research received no external funding.

Institutional Review Board Statement: Not applicable.

Informed Consent Statement: Not applicable.

References

1. Etemad-Shahidi, Y.; Qallandar, O.B.; Evenden, J.; Alifui-Segbaya, F.; Ahmed, K.E. Accuracy of 3-Dimensionally Printed Full-Arch Dental Models: A Systematic Review. *J. Clin. Med.* **2020**, *9*, 3357. [CrossRef]
2. Abduo, J.; Lyons, K.; Bennamoun, M. Trends in computer-aided manufacturing in prosthodontics: A review of the available streams. *Int. J. Dent.* **2014**, *2014*, 783948. [CrossRef] [PubMed]
3. Stansbury, J.W.; Idacavage, M.J. 3D printing with polymers: Challenges among expanding options and opportunities. *Dent. Mater.* **2015**, *32*, 54–64. [CrossRef]
4. Cheng, C.-W.; Ye, S.-Y.; Chien, C.-H.; Chen, C.-J.; Papaspyridakos, P.; Ko, C.-C. Randomised clinical trial of a conventional and a digital workflow for the fabrication of interim crowns: An evaluation of treatment efficiency, fit, and the effect of clinician experience. *J. Prosthet. Dent.* **2020**, *125*, 73–81. [CrossRef]
5. Braian, M.; Jimbo, R.; Wennerberg, A. Production tolerance of additive manufactured polymeric objects for clinical applications. *Dent. Mater.* **2016**, *32*, 853–861. [CrossRef] [PubMed]
6. Dietrich, C.A.; Ender, A.; Baumgartner, S.; Mehl, A.A. validation study of reconstructed rapid prototyping models produced by two technologies. *Angle Orthod.* **2017**, *87*, 782–787. [CrossRef] [PubMed]
7. Alghazzawi, T.F. Advancements in CAD/CAM technology: Options for practical implementation. *J. Prosthodont. Res.* **2016**, *60*, 72–84. [CrossRef]
8. Dawood, A.; Marti, B.M.; Sauret-jackson, V.; Darwood, A. 3D printing in dentistry. *Br. Dent. J.* **2015**, *219*, 521–529. [CrossRef] [PubMed]
9. Alifui-Segbaya, F. Biomedical photopolymers in 3D printing. *Rapid Prototyp. J.* **2019**, *26*, 437–444. [CrossRef]
10. Tahayeri, A.; Morgan, M.; Fugolin, A.P.; Bompolaki, D.; Athirasala, A.; Pfeifer, C.S.; Ferracane, J.L.; Bertassoni, L.E. 3D printed versus conventionally cured provisional crown and bridge dental materials. *Dent. Mater.* **2018**, *34*, 192–200. [CrossRef]
11. Joda, T.; Matthisson, L.; Zitzmann, N.U. Impact of Aging on the Accuracy of 3D-Printed Dental Models: An In Vitro Investigation. *J. Clin. Med.* **2020**, *9*, 1436. [CrossRef]
12. Sabbah, A.; Romanos, G.; Delgado-Ruiz, R. Impact of Layer Thickness and Storage Time on the Properties of 3D-Printed Dental Dies. *Materials* **2021**, *14*, 509. [CrossRef]
13. Ahmed, K.E.; Whitters, J.; Ju, X.; Pierce, S.G.; MacLeod, C.N.; Murray, C.A. A proposed methodology to assess the accuracy of 3d scanners and casts and monitor tooth wear progression in patients. *Int. J. Prosthodont.* **2016**, *29*, 514–521. [CrossRef]
14. Aly, P.; Mohsen, C. Comparison of the Accuracy of Three-Dimensional Printed Casts, Digital, and Conventional Casts: An In Vitro Study. *Eur. J. Dent.* **2020**, *14*, 189–193. [CrossRef]
15. Jin, S.J.; Kim, D.Y.; Kim, J.H.; Kim, W.C. Accuracy of Dental Replica Models Using Photopolymer Materials in Additive Manufacturing: In Vitro Three-Dimensional Evaluation. *J. Prosthodont.* **2019**, *28*, e557–e562. [CrossRef] [PubMed]
16. Papaspyridakos, P.; Chen, Y.-W.; Alshawaf, B.; Kang, K.; Finkelman, M.; Chronopoulos, V.; Weber, H.-P. Digital workflow: In vitro accuracy of 3D printed casts generated from complete-arch digital implant scans. *J. Prosthet. Dent.* **2020**, *124*, 589–593. [CrossRef]
17. Yousef, H.; Harris, B.T.; Elathamna, E.N.; Morton, D.; Lin, W.S. Effect of additive manufacturing process and storage condition on the dimensional accuracy and stability of 3D-printed dental casts. *J. Prosthet. Dent.* **2021**. [CrossRef] [PubMed]
18. Wan Hassan, W.N.; Yusoff, Y.; Mardi, N.A. Comparison of reconstructed rapid prototyping models produced by 3-dimensional printing and conventional stone models with different degrees of crowding. *Am. J. Orthod. Dentofacial. Orthop.* **2017**, *151*, 209–218. [CrossRef]
19. Dong, T.; Wang, X.; Xia, L.; Yuan, L.; Ye, N.; Fang, B. Accuracy of different tooth surfaces on 3D printed dental models: Orthodontic perspective. *BMC Oral Health* **2020**, *20*, 340. [CrossRef] [PubMed]
20. Revilla-León, M.; Subramanian, S.G.; Att, W.; Krishnamurthy, V.R. Analysis of Different Illuminance of the Room Lighting Condition on the Accuracy (Trueness and Precision) of An Intraoral Scanner. *J. Prosthodont.* **2021**, *30*, 157–162. [CrossRef]
21. Revilla-León, M.; Jiang, P.; Sadeghpour, M.; Piedra-Cascón, W.; Zandinejad, A.; Özcan, M.; Krishnamurthy, V.R. Intraoral digital scans-Part 1: Influence of ambient scanning light conditions on the accuracy (trueness and precision) of different intraoral scanners. *J. Prosthet. Dent.* **2020**, *124*, 372–378. [CrossRef]
22. Kim, Y.H.; Han, S.-S.; Choi, Y.J.; Woo, C.-W. Linear Accuracy of Full-Arch Digital Models Using Four Different Scanning Methods: An In Vitro Study Using a Coordinate Measuring Machine. *Appl. Sci.* **2020**, *10*, 2741. [CrossRef]
23. Resende, C.C.D.; Barbosa, T.A.Q.; Moura, G.F.; Tavares, L.D.N.; Rizzante, F.A.P.; George, F.M.; Neves, F.D.D.; Mendonça, G. Influence of operator experience, scanner type, and scan size on 3D scans. *J. Prosthet. Dent.* **2021**, *125*, 294–299. [CrossRef] [PubMed]
24. Lim, J.H.; Mangal, U.; Nam, N.E.; Choi, S.H.; Shim, J.S.; Kim, J.E. A Comparison of Accuracy of Different Dental Restorative Materials between Intraoral Scanning and Conventional Impression-Taking: An In Vitro Study. *Materials* **2021**, *14*, 2060. [CrossRef]

25. Kim, S.Y.; Shin, Y.S.; Jung, H.D.; Hwang, C.J.; Baik, H.S.; Cha, J.Y. Precision and trueness of dental models manufactured with different 3-dimensional printing techniques. *Am. J. Orthod. Dentofacial. Orthop.* **2018**, *153*, 144–153. [CrossRef] [PubMed]
26. Hazeveld, A.; Huddleston Slater, J.J.R.; Ren, Y. Accuracy and reproducibility of dental replica models reconstructed by different rapid prototyping techniques. *Am. J. Orthod. Dentofacial. Orthop.* **2014**, *145*, 108–115. [CrossRef]
27. Zhang, Z.-C.; Li, P.-l.; Chu, F.-T.; Shen, G. Influence of the three-dimensional printing technique and printing layer thickness on model accuracy. *J. Orofac. Orthop.* **2019**, *80*, 194–204. [CrossRef] [PubMed]
28. Nestler, N.; Wesemann, C.; Spies, B.C.; Beuer, F.; Bumann, A. Dimensional accuracy of extrusion- and photopolymerisation-based 3D printers: In vitro study comparing printed casts. *J. Prosthet. Dent.* **2020**, *125*, 103–110. [CrossRef]
29. Lin, C.-H.; Lin, Y.-M.; Lai, Y.-L.; Lee, S.-Y. Mechanical properties, accuracy, and cytotoxicity of UV-polymerized 3D printing resins composed of Bis-EMA, UDMA, and TEGDMA. *J. Prosthet. Dent.* **2020**, *123*, 349–354. [CrossRef]
30. Reymus, M.; Lümkemann, N.; Stawarczyk, B. 3D-printed material for temporary restorations: Impact of print layer thickness and post-curing method on degree of conversion. *Int. J. Comput. Dent.* **2019**, *22*, 231–237.
31. Jang, Y.; Sim, J.Y.; Park, J.K.; Kim, W.C.; Kim, H.Y.; Kim, J.H. Evaluation of the marginal and internal fit of a single crown fabricated based on a three-dimensional printed model. *J. Adv. Prosthodont.* **2018**, *10*, 367–373. [CrossRef]
32. Contrepois, M.; Soenen, A.; Bartala, M.; Laviole, O. Marginal adaptation of ceramic crowns: A systematic review. *J. Prosthet. Dent.* **2013**, *110*, 447–454.e10. [CrossRef] [PubMed]
33. McLean, J.W.; von Fraunhofer, J.A. The estimation of cement film thickness by an in vivo technique. *Br. Dent. J.* **1971**, *131*, 107–111. [CrossRef] [PubMed]
34. Luthardt, R.G.; Kühmstedt, P.; Walter, M.H. A new method for the computer-aided evaluation of three-dimensional changes in gypsum materials. *Dent. Mater.* **2003**, *19*, 19–24. [CrossRef]

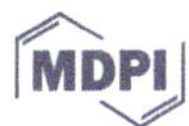

Article

Evaluation of Dimensional Changes during Postcuring of a Three-Dimensionally Printed Denture Base According to the Curing Time and the Time of Removal of the Support Structure: An In Vitro Study

Re-Mee Doh [1,†], Jong-Eun Kim [2,†], Na-Eun Nam [3], Seung-Ho Shin [3], Jung-Hwa Lim [3] and June-Sung Shim [2,*]

[1] Department of Advanced General Dentistry, Dankook University College of Dentistry, Dandae-ro 119, Dongnam-gu, Cheonan 31116, Korea; remeedoh@dankook.ac.kr
[2] Department of Prosthodontics, College of Dentistry, Yonsei University, Yonsei-ro 50-1, Seodaemun-gu, Seoul 03722, Korea; gomyou@yuhs.ac
[3] Department of Prosthodontics, Oral Research Science Center, BK21 PLUS Project, Yonsei University College of Dentistry, Yonsei-ro 50-1, Seodaemun-gu, Seoul 03722, Korea; jennynam90@yuhs.ac (N.-E.N.); shin506@prostholabs.com (S.-H.S.); erin0313@prostholabs.com (J.-H.L.)
* Correspondence: jfshim@yuhs.ac; Tel.: +82-2-2228-3157
† These authors contributed equally to this work as first authors.

Featured Application: In the postcuring process after 3D printing, a dimensional change occurs, and when the postcuring process is performed after the support structure is removed, the change occurs more significantly.

Abstract: This study attempted to determine the dimensional stability of maxillary and mandibular edentulous denture bases constructed using three-dimensional (3D) printing systems based on stereolithography and digital light processing according to the postcuring treatment time and the removal time of the support structure. Three-dimensional printing of the designed denture base file was performed using two types of 3D printing photocurable resin (standard gray resin (Formlabs) (Somerville, MA, USA) and MAZIC D resin (Vericom) (Anyang, Korea)) and their compatible 3D printers (Form3 (Formlabs) and Phrozen Shuffle (Phrozen) (Hsinchu City, Taiwan)). Different postcuring times (no postcuring, and 15, 30, 45, and 60 min) and times of removal of the support structure were set for each group. Data relating to the denture bases in all groups were obtained using 3D scanning with a tabletop scanner after postcuring. All acquired data were exported to 3D analysis software, and the dimensional changes during postcuring of the denture base were analyzed using RMSE (root-mean-square error) values. It could be confirmed that the dimensional changes increased with postcuring time, and the accuracy was higher in the maxilla than in the mandible. The accuracy was highest for the group in which the postcuring process was performed while the support structure was present.

Keywords: 3D printing; dimensional stability; support structure; postcuring

Citation: Doh, R.-M.; Kim, J.-E.; Nam, N.-E.; Shin, S.-H.; Lim, J.-H.; Shim, J.-S. Evaluation of Dimensional Changes during Postcuring of a Three-Dimensionally Printed Denture Base According to the Curing Time and the Time of Removal of the Support Structure: An In Vitro Study. *Appl. Sci.* **2021**, *11*, 10000. https://doi.org/10.3390/app112110000

Academic Editor: Kathrin Becker

Received: 9 October 2021
Accepted: 25 October 2021
Published: 26 October 2021

Publisher's Note: MDPI stays neutral with regard to jurisdictional claims in published maps and institutional affiliations.

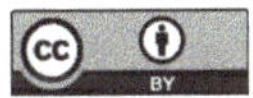

1. Introduction

Three-dimensional printing is also called additive manufacturing or rapid prototyping, and it has contributed to the popularization of digital dentistry while overcoming the limitations of subtractive machining methods based on milling or grinding [1,2]. The current methods of prosthesis production using 3D printing can overcome the limitations of subtractive manufacturing, such as reducing cutting forces due to the wear of milling tools, limitations associated with tool sizes, difficulty in manufacturing complex shapes, and material wastage. There are now wide ranges of equipment and raw materials with various prices and performances available in the market [3].

3D printers based on stereolithography (SLA) or digital light processing (DLP) are currently the most widely used in digital dentistry. These two methods are classified based on the light source and curing method, and they have the advantages of high-precision printing and excellent surface texture [2,4,5]. The use of various photopolymeric resins makes it possible to manufacture diverse types of objects, from individual trays and dental models to final prostheses such as radiographic stents, provisional crowns, record bases, and dentures [1,6–9]. The development and use of 3D printers facilitate the fabrication of custom prostheses with complex configurations. However, the processing principles of 3D printers mean that certain specific factors that are not present in conventional manufacturing methods need to be considered. The accuracy and mechanical properties of 3D printing can be affected by variables such as machine settings, output position or build angle, number of layers, and configuration of the support structure. However, the high diversity of 3D printers and materials and the heterogeneity of their combinations mean that the 3D printing process and the associated postcuring process still need to be optimized and standardized [10–14].

Postcuring is an essential step when using a photopolymer resin with an SLA or DLP printer, as it can cause improvements in mechanical or biological properties through crosslinking of unreacted monomers after processing of 3D printing materials [15,16]. Objects that have been printed by these printers are cleaned of unpolymerized residual monomers, and additional polymerization is performed using ultraviolet light (UV) produced by light-emitting diodes (LEDs) in postcuring equipment. The degree of polymerization greatly affects not only the biocompatibility and color stability of the fabricated object but also its mechanical properties and dimensional stability [14,17–19]. It is known that the lower the polymerization rate in the 3D printing process, the greater the dimensional change occurs in the postcuring step, and the shrinkage of the area directly exposed to UV light occurs a lot, which can lead to bending due to non-uniform shrinkage [20]. Minimizing errors in the production process, and especially in the 3D printing process and postcuring, can result in a more predictable prosthesis manufacturing workflow. Several studies have investigated the precision, dimensional stability, and mechanical properties using several 3D printers [11,12,21–27]. Many companies provide guidelines for the use of materials and equipment required for the 3D printing process. However, in the process of manufacturing a series of prostheses using various products as an open system, it is often difficult to follow the guidelines of the company as it is. In addition, there are no unified guidelines among companies. Users are making the process based on empirical evidence.

During the postcuring process, a dimensional change is expected because additional curing of the residual uncured resin occurs, but studies on this are lacking. In addition, the support structure that connects the bottom surface where printing starts on the 3D printer's platform and the prosthesis is essential for the 3D printing process and is thought to play a role in stabilizing the dimension of the workpiece in the subsequent postcuring process. However, to the best of our knowledge, there was no study on the effect of the removal time of the support structure in the 3D printing process. Rather, in many experiments involving 3D printers, the timing of removal of the support structure was not controlled. Studies relating to the accuracy and mechanical properties of produced samples can be divided into those where the support structure was removed after postcuring [21,27] or before postcuring [24,25] or not accurately recorded [10,12,13,25].

This study produced maxillary and mandibular edentulous denture bases using a 3D printing system based on SLA and DLP technologies, with the aim of determining the dimensional stability according to the postcuring time and the presence or absence of a support structure during postcuring. The null hypothesis was that the dimensional stability of the denture base produced by 3D printing does not differ significantly with the postcuring time, the presence or absence of a support structure during postcuring, or the arch position.

2. Materials and Methods

For designing the standard denture base, a fully edentulous maxilla and mandible reference model was selected and then scanned using a tabletop scanner (Identica T500, Medit, Seoul, Korea). After importing the scanned model data into CAD software for dental use (Exocad DentalCAD, Exocad, Darmstadt, Germany), the denture base was designed, and the designed data were exported as an STL (standard tessellation language) file (Figure 1).

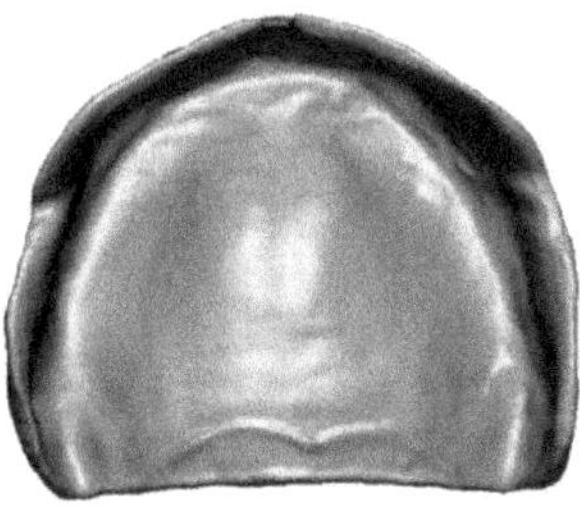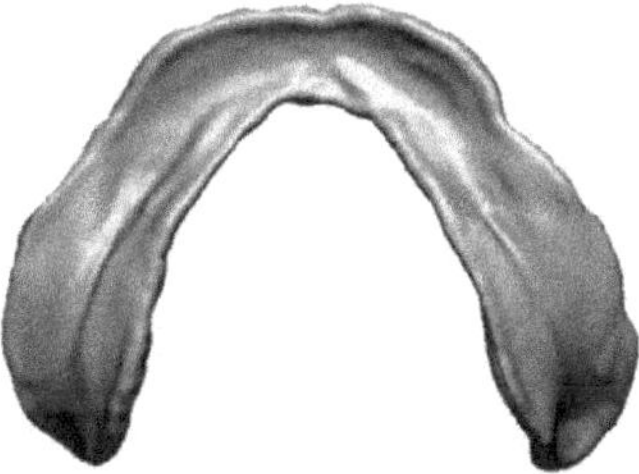

Figure 1. Designs of the experimental maxillary and mandibular denture bases.

Two types of 3D printing photocurable resin were used for the 3D printing of the design file: standard gray resin (Formlabs, Somerville, MA, USA) and MAZIC D resin (Vericom, Anyang, Korea) (Table 1). Each photocurable resin was mixed in accordance with the manufacturer's recommended mixing time using a material mixing unit (LC-3DMixer, NextDent, Soesterberg, The Netherlands) to ensure that the contents were adequately mixed prior to printing. In order to optimally three-dimensionally print the material used, slicing software and a 3D printer with settings compatible with each photocurable resin were used. For printing MAZIC D resin, support generation and mesh slicing were performed using slicing software (Chitu DLP Slicer, CBD-Tech, Guangdong, China) for 3D printing.

Table 1. The three-dimensional-printing photopolymer resins used in this study.

Product	Components	Manufacturer
Standard gray resin	75–90% methacrylic oligomers, 25–50% methacrylate monomer, 1–3% 2,4,6-trimethylbenzoyl-diphenyl-diphenyl phosphine oxide	Formlabs, Somerville, MA, USA
MAZIC D resin	88–98% ethoxylated bisphenol A dimethacrylate, 2–5% 2,4,6-trimethylbenzoyl-diphenyl-diphenyl phosphine oxide	Vericom, Anyang, Korea

A support structure was placed on the outer surface of the denture base, and the thickness of each building layer was set to 100 μm. Three-dimensional printing of the mesh file was performed using a DLP 3D printer with 24,405-nm UV LEDs in a 50-W matrix (ParaLED, Phrozen Shuffle, Phrozen, Hsinchu, Taiwan). For the standard gray resin, the support arrangement design specified by the Chitu DLP Slicer software was imported into the Preform slicer software (Formlabs, Somervill, MA, USA) to make the same arrangement, and three-dimensionally printed using a compatible SLA 3D printer with a 250-mW 405-nm UV LED (Form3, Formlabs). Each manufactured denture base was washed with 100% isopropyl alcohol for 10 min using washing equipment (TwinTornado, Medifive, Seoul, Korea) and then postcured using a postcuring device (MP100, Hebsiba, Incheon, Korea).

For the purpose of this study, the postcuring time and the removal of the support structure before the postcuring process were set differently for each group. In the no-support group, after 3D printing the denture base, the support structure was removed prior to carrying out postcuring. For the support group, postcuring was performed without removal of the support structure after printing the denture base. In addition to a control group (with no postcuring), postcuring times of 15, 30, 45, and 60 min were employed ($n = 10$ for each denture base). Data relating to the denture base in all groups were obtained using 3D scanning with a tabletop scanner after postcuring. The overall experimental workflow employed in this study is outlined in Figure 2.

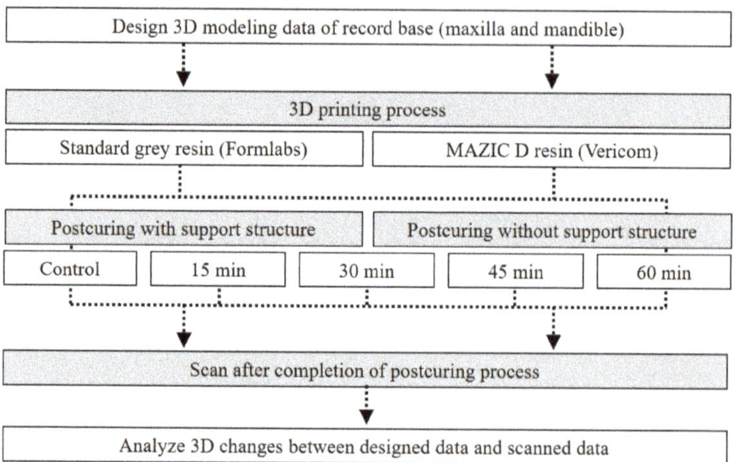

Figure 2. Flowchart of the overall experimental process of this study. The accuracy was evaluated according to the three-dimensional (3D)-printing material used, whether the support structure was removed, and the postcuring time.

All acquired data were exported to 3D analysis software (Geomagic Control X, 3D Systems, Rock Hill, SC, USA). To analyze the dimensional changes during postcuring of the denture base, the 3D modeling data and the scanned data after postcuring were compared and analyzed. The data to be compared were initially aligned using a three-point registration process and then further aligned using a best-fit algorithm. Differences between the groups were analyzed using the root-mean-square error (RMSE) values calculated as follows (1):

$$\text{RMSE} = \frac{1}{\sqrt{n}} \cdot \sqrt{\sum_{i=1}^{n}(x_{1,i} - x_{2,i})^2} \tag{1}$$

where $x_{1,i}$ is the measurement point of reference i, $x_{2,i}$ is the measurement point of scan data i, and n is the total number of points measured in each data set. The overall deviations were displayed in color maps to facilitate intuitive comparisons, assigning a deviation range of ± 500 μm and a tolerance of ± 50 μm.

Standard statistical software (SPSS Statistics, version 25.0, IBM Corporation, Armonk, NY, USA) was used for the statistical analyses. The Shapiro–Wilk test was performed to confirm that the data in each group conformed to a normal distribution. Three-way ANOVA was used to evaluate the effect of the presence or absence of a support structure during postcuring, arch position (maxilla or mandible), and postcuring time on the RMSE values between the modeling and scanned data. One-way ANOVA was used to test dimensional changes within the same arch and materials based on the postcuring time, and a post-hoc test was performed using the Bonferroni method ($\alpha = 0.05$). Differences between the support and no-support groups according to time in the same arch and the same material were analyzed using Student's *t*-test ($\alpha = 0.05$).

3. Results

The results of the three-way ANOVAs of standard gray resin and MAZIC D resin are presented in Figures 3 and 4. The three-way ANOVA of standard gray resin for the RMSE values between the modeling and scan data after the postcuring process confirmed that the dimensional changes were significantly affected by whether the support structure was removed ($F = 17.317$, $p < 0.001$), the arch position ($F = 567.555$, $p < 0.001$), and the postcuring time ($F = 9.755$, $p < 0.001$) (Figure 3). The accuracy was higher for the group in which the support structure was present during the postcuring process than for the group without support and higher for the maxilla than for the mandible. The error increased gradually with the postcuring time during the process of polymerization of the unpolymerized residual resin. However, there were no significant interactions between support removal and arch position ($F = 2.151$, $p = 0.144$), support removal and postcuring time ($F = 1.295$, $p = 0.274$), or arch position and postcuring time ($F = 0.805$, $p = 0.523$), nor between all three factors ($F = 0.268$, $p = 0.898$).

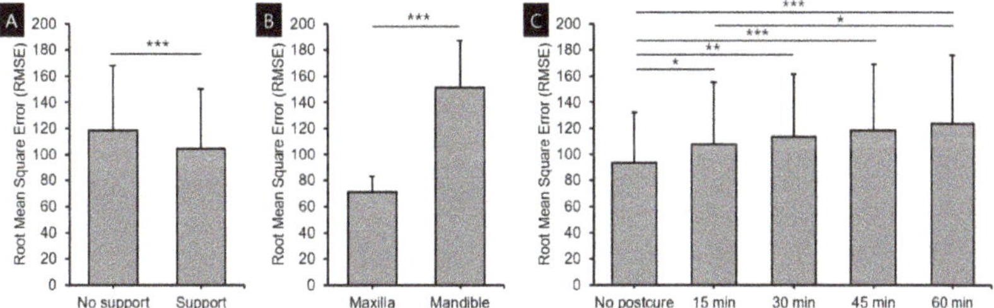

Figure 3. Three-way ANOVA results of root-mean-square error (RMSE) values for the standard gray resin specimens with respect to (**A**) whether the support structure was removed during postcuring, (**B**) arch position, and (**C**) postcuring time. Data are mean and standard deviation values. *, $p \leq 0.05$; **, $p \leq 0.01$; ***, $p \leq 0.001$.

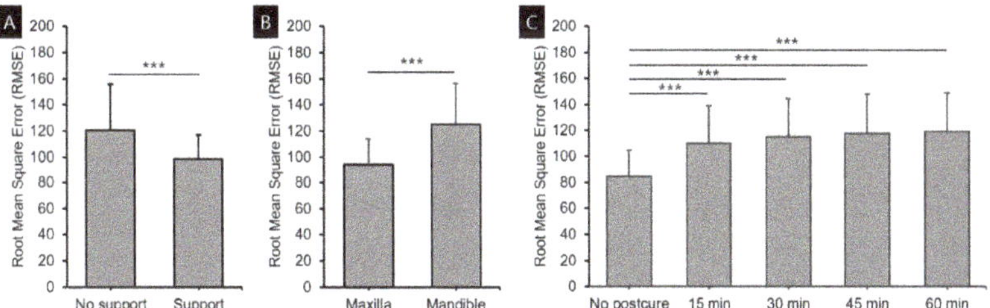

Figure 4. Three-way ANOVA results of RMSE values for the MAZIC D resin specimens with respect to (**A**) whether the support structure was removed during postcuring, (**B**) arch position, and (**C**) postcuring time. Data are mean and standard deviation values. ***, $p \leq 0.001$.

The three-way ANOVA of MAZIC D resin confirmed that the dimensional changes were significantly affected by support removal ($F = 98.774$, $p < 0.001$), arch position ($F = 191.145$, $p < 0.001$), and postcuring time ($F = 32.032$, $p < 0.001$) (Figure 4). The accuracy was highest in the group in which the support structure was present and the maxillary group, and the error increased with the postcuring time. Significant interactions were observed between support removal and arch position ($F = 66.668$, $p < 0.001$), support removal and postcuring time ($F = 8.174$, $p < 0.001$), and among all three factors ($F = 3.786$, $p = 0.006$). However, there was no significant interaction between the arch position and postcuring time ($F = 0.590$, $p = 0.670$).

Dimensional accuracy was evaluated when the same 3D printing resin was used in the same arch, and the overall results are presented in Figures 5 and 6 and in Table 2. For the maxilla base printed three-dimensionally using standard gray resin, the dimensional changes were smaller in the group in which postcuring was performed with the support structure present. The error increased with the postcuring time even in the specimen with the support structure, but the magnitude of the increase was relatively small. The error ranges in the no-support, and support groups were 58.3–83.6 µm and 58.9–72.9 µm, respectively. The accuracy differed significantly between the presence and absence of the support structure for all postcuring times, but not in the control group that did not undergo postcuring (Figure 5A). The pattern was the same in the mandible-base group printed using standard gray resin, but the accuracy was lower than in the maxillary group, with error ranges of 130.4–185.6 µm in the no-support group and 124.8–148.0 µm in the support group (Figure 5B).

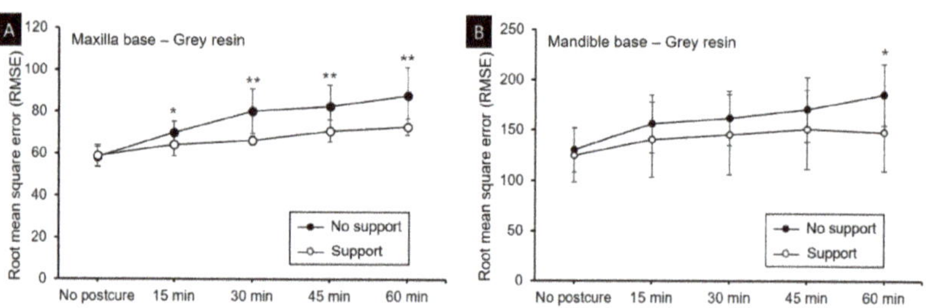

Figure 5. RMSE values during the postcuring process in the no-support and support groups using standard gray resin. (**A**) Maxilla base. (**B**) Mandible base. Data are mean and standard deviation values. *, $p \leq 0.05$; **, $p \leq 0.01$ between the no-support and support groups.

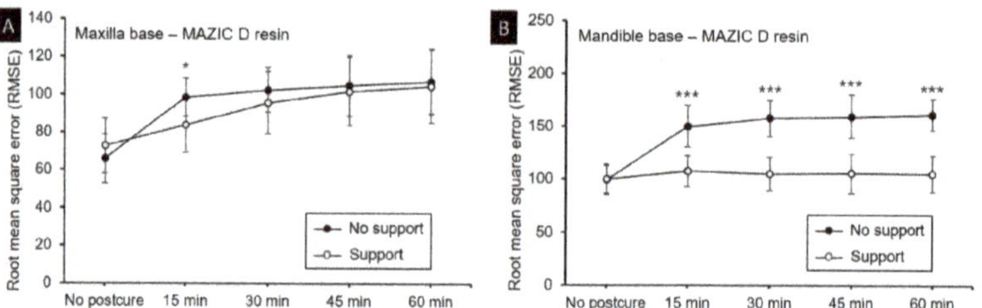

Figure 6. RMSE values during the postcuring process in the no-support and support groups using MAZIC D resin. (**A**) Maxilla base. (**B**) Mandible base. Data are mean and standard deviation values. *, $p \leq 0.05$; ***, $p \leq 0.001$ between the no-support and support groups.

Table 2. Root-mean-square error (RMSE) values for standard gray resin and MAZIC D resin specimens according to postcuring time, arch position (maxilla and mandible), and the presence or absence of a support structure. Data are mean ± standard deviation values.

			No Postcuring	15 min	30 min	45 min	60 min
Standard gray resin	Maxilla	No support	58.3 ± 4.8 [A,a]	69.8 ± 5.5 [A,ab]	80.2 ± 10.7 [A,bc]	82.6 ± 10.3 [A,c]	87.6 ± 13.8 [A,c]
		Support	58.9 ± 5.2 [A,a]	64.1 ± 5.4 [B,b]	66.2 ± 2.2 [B,bc]	70.9 ± 5.2 [B,cd]	72.9 ± 3.9 [B,d]
	Mandible	No support	130.4 ± 22.0 [A,a]	156.3 ± 29.1 [A,ab]	161.8 ± 27.0 [A,ab]	170.7 ± 32.3 [A,b]	185.6 ± 30.6 [A,b]
		Support	124.8 ± 26.9 [A,a]	140.6 ± 37.2 [A,a]	145.5 ± 40.1 [A,a]	151.0 ± 39.3 [A,a]	148.0 ± 38.8 [B,a]
MAZIC D resin	Maxilla	No support	65.8 ± 12.9 [A,a]	98.4 ± 10.3 [A,b]	102.4 ± 11.8 [A,b]	104.9 ± 16.1 [A,b]	106.7 ± 17.0 [A,b]
		Support	72.6 ± 14.6 [A,a]	83.7 ± 14.6 [B,ab]	95.6 ± 16.6 [A,b]	101.7 ± 18.2 [A,b]	104.6 ± 19.6 [A,b]
	Mandible	No support	99.6 ± 13.9 [A,a]	150.1 ± 19.8 [A,b]	157.9 ± 17.4 [A,b]	159.6 ± 20.6 [A,b]	161.3 ± 14.9 [A,b]
		Support	99.7 ± 13.0 [A,a]	107.3 ± 14.6 [B,a]	105.0 ± 15.8 [B,a]	105.4 ± 18.4 [B,a]	105.1 ± 17.1 [B,a]

Different uppercase superscript letters indicate significant differences in RMSE values within columns depending on whether or not the support structure was removed during the postcuring process. Different lowercase superscript letters indicate significant differences in RMSE values within rows according to the postcuring time.

When printing denture bases using MAZIC D resin, the dimensional changes in the no-support group were largest after the first 15 min of postcuring for both the maxillary and mandibular bases, after which there were no significant variations in the dimensional changes (Figure 6). In the maxilla group with MAZIC D resin, the dimensions changed during the postcuring process even when the support structure was present, and the errors were in the range of 72.6–104.6 μm. There was a significant difference between the no-support and support groups only after 15 min of postcuring, with a large initial dimensional change in the no-support group, but no change thereafter. It seems that the polymerization of MAZIC D resin proceeded faster than the standard gray resin (Figure 6A). In the mandible group with MAZIC D, there was no significant dimensional change when the support structure was present during the postcuring process, and the error range was 99.7–105.1 μm. There were significant differences between the no-support and support groups at all postcuring time periods other than for the control group (Figure 6B).

The qualitative overall deviation results are presented as color maps in Figures 7 and 8. The error was smallest in the control group without postcuring. In the case of the maxilla, there were positive errors in the anterior alveolar ridge area and the maxillary tuberosity area and negative errors in the center of the palate. As the postcuring time increased, the flange area of the denture base around the posterior teeth showed a pattern of increasing positive errors, and the palate area showed a pattern of increasing negative errors. In the case of the mandible, the errors were largest in the retromolar pad area, where there were positive errors. The alveolar ridge area around the lingual border and the premolar area showed negative errors. In these areas, the errors increased with the postcuring time. The groups using standard gray resin and MAZIC D resin showed similar trends (Figures 7 and 8).

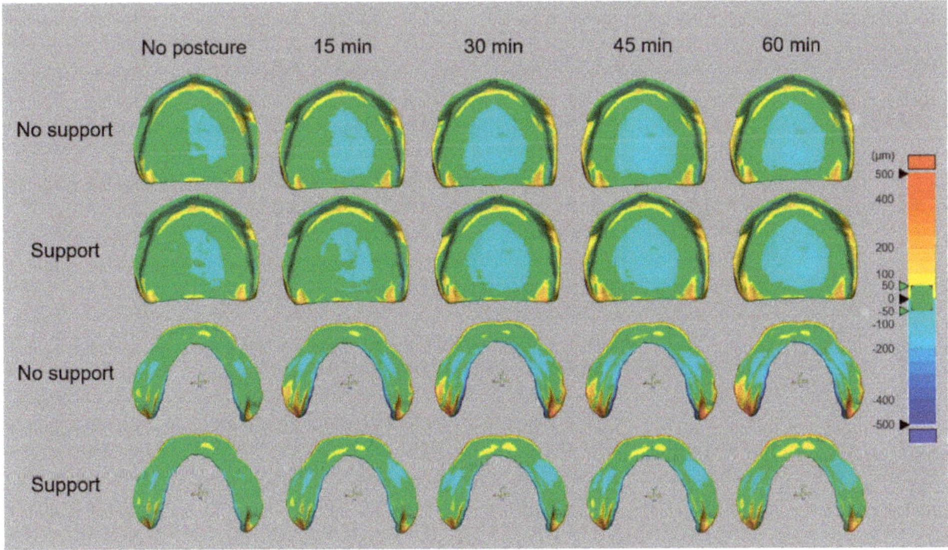

Figure 7. Overall deviations of denture bases produced using the standard gray resin and Form3 3D printer presented as color maps. Deviation range of ±500 μm and a tolerance of ±50 μm was set.

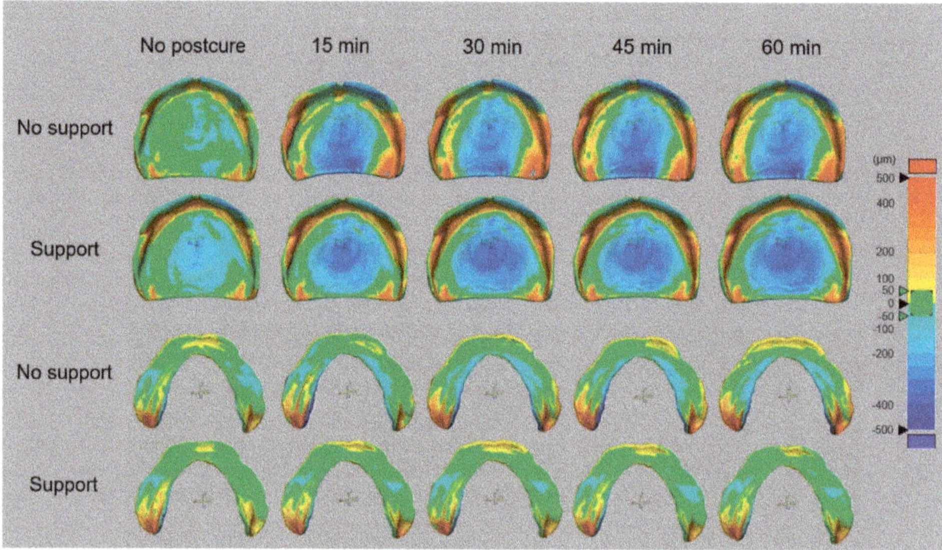

Figure 8. Overall deviations of denture bases produced using the MAZIC D resin and Phrozen Shuffle 3D printer presented as color maps. Deviation range of ±500 µm and a tolerance of ±50 µm was set.

4. Discussion

The purpose of this study was to determine the dimensional stability of maxillary and mandibular edentulous denture bases according to the postcuring time and whether the support structure is present or removed during the postcuring process after 3D printing. Denture-based samples were constructed using 3D printers with two resins, and postcuring times of 0, 15, 30, 45, and 60 min were investigated. Three-way ANOVAs showed that when using the SLA-type Form3 printer and standard gray resin or the DLP-type Phrozen Shuffle printer and MAZIC D resin, the accuracy was significantly higher when postcuring was performed with the support structure present and higher for the maxilla than the mandible. The dimensional changes gradually accumulated, and the deviations increased with the postcuring time. Therefore, the null hypothesis of this study, that there are no dimensional changes according to the removal of the support structure, arch position, and postcuring time, was rejected.

Most previous studies have found that digital dentures and record bases produced by 3D printing are highly accurate. In the present experiments, when using standard gray resin with the SLA-type Form3 printer, the error in the no-support group increased significantly with the postcuring time for both maxillary and mandibular denture bases. In the support group, there were significant changes as the postcuring time increased in the maxilla, but there were few changes in the dimension for the mandible and no significant differences according to the postcuring time (Figure 5, Table 2). Kalberer et al. [24], which was designed to remove the support structure before postcuring, is noteworthy that the accuracy was inferior in their 3D printing group, which contrasts with other studies. Those authors observed a significantly larger dimensional difference for the maxillary edentulous denture base constructed using an SLA 3D printer than for the milled type of base. They attributed this observation to the deformation of partially polymerized prostheses during demounting or to polymerization shrinkage. Their analysis results are consistent with those of the present experiments, which showed that differences in dimensional changes appeared with or without a support structure.

In both the SLA and DLP methods, the postcuring step is as important as the design and printing processes, and an insufficient postcuring time can result in dimensional changes or reduced strength due to the presence of unpolymerized resin [28]. If the output is an individual tray, insufficient postcuring may result in distortion of the tray and the impression body after obtaining the impression. In the case of a denture base, insufficient postcuring may cause issues relating to its fit, which affects the accuracy of the artificial tooth attachment due to warping of the joint, and may, in turn, lead to an overall occlusal error. In addition, even for a three-dimensionally printed model, insufficient postcuring can lead to errors in the fabrication of the prosthesis that cause serious problems [29].

In the present experiments using the MAZIC D resin and the DLP-type Phrozen Shuffle 3D printer, dimensional changes during postcuring were hardly observed in the group with the support structure present. However, in the group where the support structure was not present, a rapid change in dimensions was observed during the first 15 min of postcuring. As mentioned above, this is considered to be due to a problem with the initial polymerization rate. Additional changes may have occurred due to the presence of bulk resin in the palate area and the direction of polymerization shrinkage in this direction. The difference in the characteristics of change between standard gray resin and Mazic D resin seems to be due not only to the difference in initial polymerization due to the difference between SLA and DLP but also to the faster polymerization rate of MAZIC D resin during the postcuring period. Preventing such a dimensional change due to the presence of residual monomers requires the manufacturer's instructions to be followed exactly. However, since many CAD/CAM systems are open-source systems and due to various types of 3D printers, software, and materials being used by clinicians and laboratories, the manufacturer's instructions related to the use of standardized company equipment and resins might diverge. In addition, it should be considered that the postcuring time may vary with the values set for 3D printing devices [25].

When using MAZIC D resin and a DLP 3D printer, continuous errors were observed in the maxilla regardless of the postcuring time or presence of a support structure. The larger error for the maxilla than for the mandible was attributed to the large error in the palate area. The palate of the maxilla can play a role in maintaining the dimensional stability of the fabricated object, such as a support structure used in the 3D printing process does, but unlike the support structure, it is an area that is used without being removed. Hwang et al. [12] recently found both positive and negative errors in the maxillary palate for maxillary denture bases produced using the DLP 3D printer, which is similar results to this present experiments. Those authors attributed the geometry deviations to the 100-degree construction angle and sagging of the liquid material under its own weight. This analysis can be supported through the result that palate error is small even in the milled type manufacturing method [12,30]. In addition, in the postcuring process, since there may be a difference in the shrinkage between the part that is directly irradiated with UV light and the part that is not directly irradiated with UV light, this may cause bending and lead to an error in the denture base [20]. In this study, the average RMSE values of standard gray resin and MAZIC D resin were similar, but in the color map shown in Figure 7, it was confirmed that the overall deviation of MAZIC D resin was large. This trend was especially observed in the maxilla, and it can be confirmed through the fact that the standard deviation value of MAZIC D resin is higher than that of standard gray resin in all postcuring time periods.

Recent comparative studies found that the accuracy of 3D printing methods was equivalent to or better than those of existing milling methods [21,26,27], although inaccurate and irreproducible results have also been reported [24,25]. It is noteworthy that these studies involved various postcuring times and support-structure removal times. Those experiments applied postcuring times such as 10, 15, and 30 min, or the exact time was not recorded [10,24,25,27]. More accurate comparative experiments require the postcuring time to be properly controlled and recorded, given that this is a very important parameter.

The present study was subject to some limitations. Since the required postcuring time varies with the 3D printer, material type, and light source (e.g., its wavelength and intensity) of the postcuring device, standard guidelines cannot be determined solely from the results of this study. In addition, while two types of materials, 3D printers and denture bases with a uniform thickness, were used in the present experiments, the diversity of materials and equipment will be greater in in vivo applications, and the thickness will vary according to the type of residual ridge. Future studies involving various types of equipment, materials, layer thicknesses, and irregular shapes may provide more meaningful guidelines for the optimal conditions to use when producing prostheses using 3D printing technology.

5. Conclusions

Based on the findings of this in vitro study, the following conclusions can be drawn:

1. When using either the SLA-type Form3 printer and standard gray resin or the DLP-type Phrozen Shuffle printer and MAZIC D resin, postcuring with the support structure resulted in significantly higher accuracy than when the support structure was removed;
2. In both types of resin, it was confirmed that the output error of the maxillary denture base was lower than that of the mandible;
3. When using either the SLA-type Form3 printer and standard gray resin or the DLP-type Phrozen Shuffle printer and MAZIC D resin, dimensional changes gradually accumulated, and deviations increased with the postcuring time;
4. When using the DLP-type Phrozen Shuffle printer and MAZIC D resin, large dimensional changes occurred after the first 15 min of postcuring.

Author Contributions: Conceptualization, R.-M.D., J.-E.K. and J.-S.S.; Data curation, R.-M.D., J.-E.K., N.-E.N., S.-H.S. and J.-H.L.; Formal analysis, R.-M.D., J.-E.K., N.-E.N., S.-H.S. and J.-H.L.; Funding acquisition, R.-M.D.; Investigation, J.-E.K.; Methodology, J.-E.K., S.-H.S. and J.-H.L.; Project administration, J.-E.K.; Resources, J.-E.K. and N.-E.N.; Software, N.-E.N. and S.-H.S.; Validation, R.-M.D., S.-H.S. and J.-S.S.; Visualization, R.-M.D., J.-E.K. and J.-H.L.; Writing—original draft, R.-M.D., J.-E.K., N.-E.N. and J.-S.S.; Writing—review and editing, R.-M.D., J.-E.K., N.-E.N., S.-H.S., J.-H.L. and J.-S.S. All authors have read and agreed to the published version of the manuscript.

Funding: This work was supported by Basic Science Research Program through the National Research Foundation of Korea (NRF), funded by the Ministry of Science and ICT (NRF-2019R1G1A1085775).

Institutional Review Board Statement: Not applicable.

Informed Consent Statement: Not applicable.

Data Availability Statement: The data presented in this study are available on request from the corresponding author.

Conflicts of Interest: The authors declare no conflict of interest.

References

1. Barazanchi, A.; Li, K.C.; Al-Amleh, B.; Lyons, K.; Waddell, J.N. Additive technology: Update on current materials and applications in dentistry. *J. Prosthodont.* **2017**, *26*, 156–163. [CrossRef] [PubMed]
2. Kessler, A.; Hickel, R.; Reymus, M. 3d printing in dentistry-state of the art. *Oper. Dent.* **2020**, *45*, 30–40. [CrossRef]
3. Abduo, J.; Lyons, K.; Bennamoun, M. Trends in computer-aided manufacturing in prosthodontics: A review of the available streams. *Int. J. Dent.* **2014**, *2014*, 783948. [CrossRef]
4. Dawood, A.; Marti Marti, B.; Sauret-Jackson, V.; Darwood, A. 3d printing in dentistry. *Br. Dent. J.* **2015**, *219*, 521–529. [CrossRef] [PubMed]
5. Revilla-Leon, M.; Fogarty, R.; Barrington, J.J.; Zandinejad, A.; Ozcan, M. Influence of scan body design and digital implant analogs on implant replica position in additively manufactured casts. *J. Prosthet. Dent.* **2020**, *124*, 202–210. [CrossRef]
6. Alharbi, N.; Wismeijer, D.; Osman, R.B. Additive manufacturing techniques in prosthodontics: Where do we currently stand? A critical review. *Int. J. Prosthodont.* **2017**, *30*, 474–484. [CrossRef]
7. Jurado, C.A.; Tsujimoto, A.; Alhotan, A.; Villalobos-Tinoco, J.; AlShabib, A. Digitally fabricated immediate complete dentures: Case reports of milled and printed dentures. *Int. J. Prosthodont.* **2020**, *33*, 232–241. [CrossRef]
8. Stansbury, J.W.; Idacavage, M.J. 3d printing with polymers: Challenges among expanding options and opportunities. *Dent. Mater.* **2016**, *32*, 54–64. [CrossRef]
9. Van Noort, R. The future of dental devices is digital. *Dent. Mater.* **2012**, *28*, 3–12. [CrossRef] [PubMed]
10. Alharbi, N.; Osman, R.; Wismeijer, D. Effects of build direction on the mechanical properties of 3d-printed complete coverage interim dental restorations. *J. Prosthet. Dent.* **2016**, *115*, 760–767. [CrossRef]

11. Alharbi, N.; Osman, R.B.; Wismeijer, D. Factors influencing the dimensional accuracy of 3d-printed full-coverage dental restorations using stereolithography technology. *Int. J. Prosthodont.* **2016**, *29*, 503–510. [CrossRef]
12. Hwang, H.J.; Lee, S.J.; Park, E.J.; Yoon, H.I. Assessment of the trueness and tissue surface adaptation of cad-cam maxillary denture bases manufactured using digital light processing. *J. Prosthet. Dent.* **2019**, *121*, 110–117. [CrossRef]
13. Osman, R.B.; Alharbi, N.; Wismeijer, D. Build angle: Does it influence the accuracy of 3d-printed dental restorations using digital light-processing technology? *Int. J. Prosthodont.* **2017**, *30*, 182–188. [CrossRef]
14. Revilla-Leon, M.; Ozcan, M. Additive manufacturing technologies used for processing polymers: Current status and potential application in prosthetic dentistry. *J. Prosthodont.* **2019**, *28*, 146–158. [CrossRef]
15. Fuh, J.Y.H.; Lu, L.; Tan, C.C.; Shen, Z.X.; Chew, S. Processing and characterising photo-sensitive polymer in the rapid prototyping process. *J. Mater. Process. Technol.* **1999**, *89–90*, 211–217. [CrossRef]
16. Cheah, C.M.; Nee, A.Y.C.; Fuh, J.Y.H.; Lu, L.; Choo, Y.S.; Miyazawa, T. Characteristics of photopolymeric material used in rapid prototypes part i. Mechanical properties in the green state. *J. Mater. Process. Technol.* **1997**, *67*, 41–45. [CrossRef]
17. Dos Santos, R.L.; de Sampaio, G.A.; de Carvalho, F.G.; Pithon, M.M.; Guenes, G.M.; Alves, P.M. Influence of degree of conversion on the biocompatibility of different composites in vivo. *J. Adhes. Dent.* **2014**, *16*, 15–20. [CrossRef] [PubMed]
18. Moldovan, M.; Balazsi, R.; Soanca, A.; Roman, A.; Sarosi, C.; Prodan, D.; Vlassa, M.; Cojocaru, I.; Saceleanu, V.; Cristescu, I. Evaluation of the degree of conversion, residual monomers and mechanical properties of some light-cured dental resin composites. *Materials* **2019**, *12*, 2109. [CrossRef] [PubMed]
19. Reymus, M.; Lumkemann, N.; Stawarczyk, B. 3D-printed material for temporary restorations: Impact of print layer thickness and post-curing method on degree of conversion. *Int. J. Comput. Dent.* **2019**, *22*, 231–237. [PubMed]
20. Wu, D.; Zhao, Z.; Zhang, Q.; Qi, H.J.; Fang, D. Mechanics of shape distortion of DLP 3D printed structures during UV post-curing. *Soft Matter* **2019**, *15*, 6151–6159. [CrossRef] [PubMed]
21. Bae, E.J.; Jeong, I.D.; Kim, W.C.; Kim, J.H. A comparative study of additive and subtractive manufacturing for dental restorations. *J. Prosthet. Dent.* **2017**, *118*, 187–193. [CrossRef]
22. Chen, H.; Yang, X.; Chen, L.; Wang, Y.; Sun, Y. Application of fdm three-dimensional printing technology in the digital manufacture of custom edentulous mandible trays. *Sci. Rep.* **2016**, *6*, 19207. [CrossRef]
23. Eftekhar Ashtiani, R.; Nasiri Khanlar, L.; Mahshid, M.; Moshaverinia, A. Comparison of dimensional accuracy of conventionally and digitally manufactured intracoronal restorations. *J. Prosthet. Dent.* **2018**, *119*, 233–238. [CrossRef] [PubMed]
24. Kalberer, N.; Mehl, A.; Schimmel, M.; Muller, F.; Srinivasan, M. Cad-cam milled versus rapidly prototyped (3d-printed) complete dentures: An in vitro evaluation of trueness. *J. Prosthet. Dent.* **2019**, *121*, 637–643. [CrossRef]
25. Lee, S.; Hong, S.J.; Paek, J.; Pae, A.; Kwon, K.R.; Noh, K. Comparing accuracy of denture bases fabricated by injection molding, cad/cam milling, and rapid prototyping method. *J. Adv. Prosthodont.* **2019**, *11*, 55–64. [CrossRef] [PubMed]
26. Reyes, A.; Turkyilmaz, I.; Prihoda, T.J. Accuracy of surgical guides made from conventional and a combination of digital scanning and rapid prototyping techniques. *J. Prosthet. Dent.* **2015**, *113*, 295–303. [CrossRef]
27. Shim, J.S.; Kim, J.E.; Jeong, S.H.; Choi, Y.J.; Ryu, J.J. Printing accuracy, mechanical properties, surface characteristics, and microbial adhesion of 3d-printed resins with various printing orientations. *J. Prosthet. Dent.* **2020**, *124*, 468–475. [CrossRef]
28. Fehling, A.W.; Hesby, R.A.; Pelleu, G.B., Jr. Dimensional stability of autopolymerizing acrylic resin impression trays. *J. Prosthet. Dent.* **1986**, *55*, 592–597. [CrossRef]
29. Joda, T.; Matthisson, L.; Zitzmann, N.U. Impact of aging on the accuracy of 3d-printed dental models: An in vitro investigation. *J. Clin. Med.* **2020**, *9*, 1436. [CrossRef]
30. Yoon, S.N.; Oh, K.C.; Lee, S.J.; Han, J.S.; Yoon, H.I. Tissue surface adaptation of cad-cam maxillary and mandibular complete denture bases manufactured by digital light processing: A clinical study. *J. Prosthet. Dent.* **2020**, *124*, 682–689. [CrossRef]

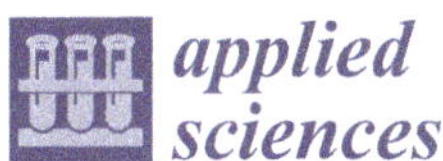 *applied sciences*

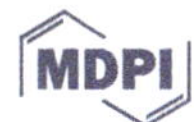

Communication

Implementation of Fused Filament Fabrication in Dentistry

Jörg Lüchtenborg, Felix Burkhardt, Julian Nold, Severin Rothlauf, Christian Wesemann, Stefano Pieralli, Gregor Wemken, Siegbert Witkowski and Benedikt C. Spies *

Department of Prosthetic Dentistry, Center for Dental Medicine, Faculty of Medicine, University of Freiburg, Hugstetter Str. 55, 79106 Freiburg, Germany; joerg.luechtenborg@uniklinik-freiburg.de (J.L.); felix.burkhardt@uniklinik-freiburg.de (F.B.); julian.nold@uniklinik-freiburg.de (J.N.); severin.rothlauf@uniklinik-freiburg.de (S.R.); christian.wesemann@uniklinik-freiburg.de (C.W.); stefano.pieralli@uniklinik-freiburg.de (S.P.); gregor.wemken@uniklinik-freiburg.de (G.W.); siegbert.witkowski@uniklinik-freiburg.de (S.W.)
* Correspondence: benedikt.spies@uniklinik-freiburg.de

Abstract: Additive manufacturing is becoming an increasingly important technique for the production of dental restorations and assistive devices. The most commonly used systems are based on vat polymerization, e.g., stereolithography (SLA) and digital light processing (DLP). In contrast, fused filament fabrication (FFF), also known under the brand name fused deposition modeling (FDM), is rarely applied in the dental field. This might be due to the reduced accuracy and resolution of FFF compared to vat polymerization. However, the use of FFF in the dental sector seems very promising for in-house production since it presents a cost-effective and straight forward method. The manufacturing of nearly ready-to-use parts with only minimal post-processing can be considered highly advantageous. Therefore, the objective was to implement FFF in a digital dental workflow. The present report demonstrates the production of surgical guides for implant insertion by FFF. Furthermore, a novel approach using a temperature-sensitive filament for bite registration plates holds great promise for a simplified workflow. In combination with a medical-grade filament, a multi-material impression tray was printed for optimized impression taking of edentulous patients. Compared to the conventional way, the printed thermoplastic material is pleasant to model and can allow clean and fast work on the patient.

Keywords: additive manufacturing; 3D printing; fused filament fabrication; fused deposition modeling; digital workflow; dentistry

Citation: Lüchtenborg, J.; Burkhardt, F.; Nold, J.; Rothlauf, S.; Wesemann, C.; Pieralli, S.; Wemken, G.; Witkowski, S.; Spies, B.C. Implementation of Fused Filament Fabrication in Dentistry . *Appl. Sci.* **2021** , *11* , 6444 . https://doi.org/10.3390/app11146444

Academic Editor: Kathrin Becker

Received: 4 June 2021
Accepted: 11 July 2021
Published: 13 July 2021

Publisher's Note: MDPI stays neutral with regard to jurisdictional claims in published maps and institutional affiliations.

1. Introduction

The development of computer-aided design and manufacturing (CAD-CAM) has facilitated manufacturing in dental laboratories. In combination with subtractive manufacturing ("milling/grinding"), reliable results and increased productivity can be achieved [1]. However, subtractive manufacturing has the disadvantage of high material loss and equipment wear. In addition, the manufactured parts can exhibit stress-related defects [2]. In contrast, with additive manufacturing (AM), components can be manufactured by adding material. This technology, also known as tool-less manufacturing technology, shows minimal wear and provides a greater degree of utilization of the feedstock material.

In AM, the virtual objects are digitally cut into layers prior to the manufacturing process. Subsequently, the virtual object is transformed into a solid component by depositing material layer by layer [3].

Currently, additive processes based on vat-polymerization, in particular stereolithography (SLA) and digital light processing (DLP) systems, are mainly used in dentistry [4,5]. These processes are based on the local light polymerization of a photosensitive resin. While the SLA process works with a laser for polymerization [6], DLP systems operate with a projector, which allows an entire layer to be exposed at the same time. This makes production time independent of the surface area covered by the object(s) and enables time-efficient production. After printing, both processes require washing of the object to remove the resin adhering to the surface. To obtain the final material properties, further post-processing by additional light-curing is necessary, which leads to the final crosslinking of the polymers [7,8]. However, post-processing equipment, consumables, such as isopropanol for the cleaning step, and requirements for occupational safety increase the costs. The use of photosensitive resin as feedstock material also requires special precautions and trained personnel to ensure adequate printing results. Especially in the case of medical products, regulations must be strictly followed during the entire manufacturing process. Therefore, a cost-efficient process with a straight-forward workflow that offers facile handling of materials and little post-processing appears promising. Thereby regulatory compliance is alleviated and the barrier to entry for the user is lowered.

Fused filament fabrication (FFF), which is also known by its trademark fused deposition modeling (FDM), represents a simplistic and low-cost method of additive manufacturing (AM). Invented in 1989 [9], the FFF process has experienced strong growth since the original patents began to expire from 2009 onwards. Today, both industrial customers and private users are stimulating the market. New FFF printers are available for a low budget, and the choice of materials is steadily increasing.

In the FFF process, a thermoplastic filament is fed to a heated nozzle. This is where the material is melted, and as the nozzle moves layer by layer in the x and y directions along the geometry, the material is deposited [10]. Apart from possible support structures for steep projections, which have to be removed, no post-processing is required and the parts can be used immediately. The simplicity makes the process very attractive, as evidenced by its widespread use.

However, FFF suffers from limited mechanical properties in build direction due to incomplete fusion of deposited strands and higher surface roughness [11]. Until now, SLA/DLP has been mainly used in dentistry, due to its superior accuracy and mechanical properties compared to FFF. Nevertheless, non-load-bearing medical devices and assistive devices with reduced accuracy requirements present a huge potential for FFF in dentistry.

2. Applied FFF Materials in Dentistry

FFF has a huge variety of available feedstock materials. Standard materials are filaments made of semi-crystalline thermoplastics such as the most commonly used polylactic acid (PLA) and the second group of amorphous polymers like (1) acrylonitrile-butadiene-styrene copolymers (ABS), (2) polycarbonates (PC), (3) polyethylene terephthalate glycol (PETG), and (4) water-soluble materials for support structures like polyvinyl alcohol (PVA) [12].

For medical use, filaments are available that are certified for short-term contact with skin and body fluids, such as polyphenylsulfone (PPSU) [13]. Surgical guides for oral implant insertion and bone-like models are made of a biocompatible filament made from a compound of polyamide-polyolefin and cellulose (PAPC) [14]. In addition, the manufacturing of polyetherketons like PEEK [15] with FFF printers for use in craniomaxillofacial implants is being evaluated [16–18]. Other filaments are certified as medical device class 1, which are products for the temporary use in the body and a low degree of invasiveness, like PETG [19], Polycaprocalactone (PCL), and poly(lactic-co-glycolic acid) (PLGA) filaments [20].

Currently, the most common application of FFF in dentistry is the production of dental models based on intraoral scans (Figure 1). Although models made by FFF are considered to have lower precision and trueness compared to SLA and DLP systems, they meet the requirement for many dental sectors [21,22]. For example, orthodontic models require a lower accuracy than models made for the manufacturing of prosthetic restorations. Low material and equipment costs and nearly ready-to-use models without post-processing make FFF economically attractive. The model shown in Figure 1 was manufactured by using a lignin-based filament (Greentec Pro, Extrudr FD3D GmbH, Lauterach, Austria) with a material cost of approximately 1 €. The printing time was comparable to SLA systems, but with no need for post-processing procedures and reduced material costs up to 80%. Additionally, other materials such as gypsum-containing filaments [23,24] can be used to produce dental models, which can also be used for thermoforming of splints.

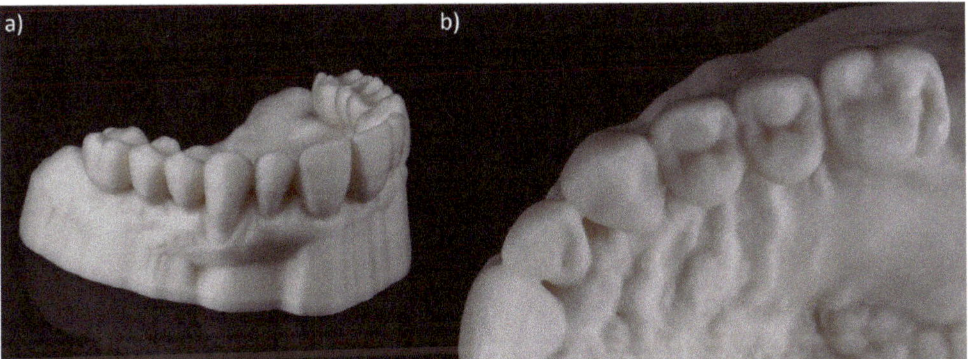

Figure 1. (**a**) Dental model of the upper jaw manufactured by fused filament fabrication (FFF), (**b**) Detailed view of highly accurate tooth structures.

Another innovative application using FFF presents the manufacturing of customized impression trays [25,26] (Figure 2a). The utilized filament (Trayfill, Berhnardt Kunstoffverarbeitungs GmbH, Berlin, Germany) is a certified medical device class 1 and withstands autoclavation [27]. This tray was printed with material costs of about 1.70 € and was therefore highly cost-effective. In order to verify the fulfillment of the required accuracy, a comparison of the STL file and the printed part was performed. Therefore, the impression tray was digitized (Keyence VL 500, Keyence, Osaka Japan) and a best-fit analysis (Geomagic Control X, 3D Systems, Inc., Rock Hill, AC, USA) was conducted (Figure 2b.) The obtained results revealed negative deviations of approximately 0.9 mm in the areas of the tuber maxillae and positive deviations of 0.2 mm in the palatal area.

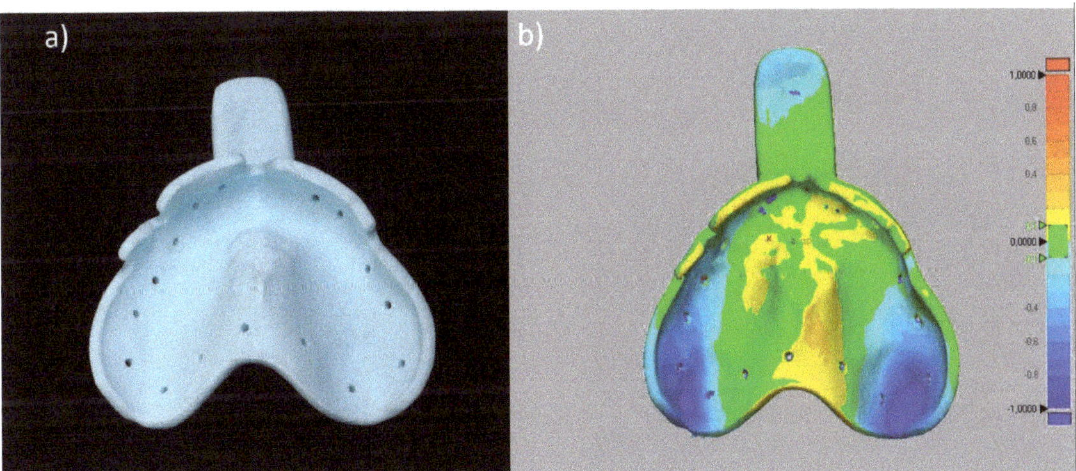

Figure 2. (**a**) Customized impression tray fabricated by means of FFF (Filament: Trayfill), (**b**) Heatmap indicating the deviation between STL file and tray.

3. Novel Approaches of FFF in Dentistry

3.1. Thermoplastic Filament for Bite Registration

Using FFF in combination with a temperature-sensitive material, a novel approach for bite registration seems to be beneficial for both the patient and the dentist. In the conventional workflow, a bite registration is performed using base plates made of light-curing acrylic and attached wax walls. The wax bite blocks are adjusted on the patient according to functional and esthetic aspects in order to convey the relation of the jaws to the dental technician. Today, based on an intraoral scan, the base plates can be digitally designed and additively manufactured using FFF in a simple and cost-effective manner. The use of a temperature-sensitive filament (Thibra3D Skulpt, Formfutura, Nijmegen, The Netherlands) allows adjustments to be made to the printed material instead of wax bite blocks. For this purpose, the printed material is heated in a hot water bath, with an alcohol burner or a hot air gun. The printed filament has a low working temperature of 70 °C, which is ideal for modeling. It can be processed unlimitedly after 3D printing and also enables the further application of the thermoplastic material. The filament is not yet classified as a medical device but ongoing cytotoxicity tests reveal promising results. The presented feasibility test (Figure 3) aimed to demonstrate the use of a temperature-sensitive filament in the dental workflow. Compared to the conventional adjustment of wax, this material is pleasant to model and holds great promise for clean and fast work on the patient.

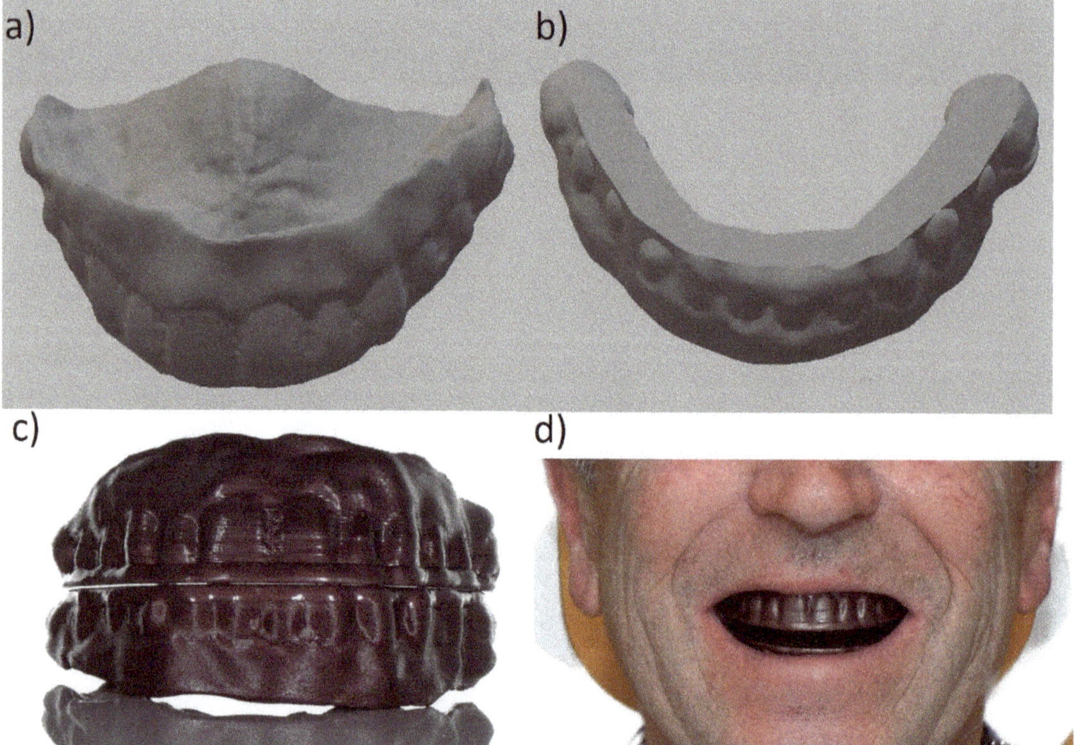

Figure 3. (**a**) STL model of the upper jaw with a flat contact surface, (**b**) STL model of the lower jaw with a flat contact surface, (**c**) bite plates manufactured by FFF (**d**) fitting of the bite plates.

To further reduce treatment time on the patient, the jaw relation of existing prostheses can be implemented in the digital workflow. In the presented case (Figure 3), the intraoral implant scans (TRIOS 4, 3Shape, Copenhagen, Denmark) of the upper and lower jaw were the basis for the design of the registration plates. By utilizing the existing screw-retained antagonistic prosthesis, a buccal scan was taken to obtain a preliminary bite registration. An automated tooth set-up (Zirkonzahn, Gais, Italy) was integrated into the CAD of the base plates, which allowed the first visualization of a potential tooth set-up. In addition, a "Plane Cut" was inserted in the occlusal plane in the Meshmixer software (Autodesk, Mill Valley, CA, USA) so that the upper and lower jaw had a flat contact surface as known from the conventional procedure (Figure 3a,b). The final designed base plates were subsequently 3D printed with the Prusa i3 (Prusa, Prague, Czech Republic) at a printing temperature of 205 °C using the previously described temperature-sensitive filament (1.75 mm). Only minimal post-processing was needed to obtain the final bite plates.

On the patient, the bite planes were inspected and slightly adjusted after heating in a water bath (Figure 3c,d). Finally, the bite plates were attached to each other by heating the occlusal surface with a hot instrument, after which the guides were removed from the mouth as a pair.

3.2. Dual Material Customized Impression Trays

Another use case for FFF in dentistry is the additive manufacturing of customized impression trays. While digital impressions present sufficient accuracy for fixed dental prostheses [28,29], the acquisition of moving areas e.g., the alveolar mucosa in the vestibule, is still associated with limitations. These areas are especially important for the retention of prostheses for edentulous patients. In a conventional workflow, impression taking is split into two steps. Before using the main impression material e.g., a thermoplastic compound material is manually applied to the rim of an individualized impression tray and intraorally adjusted by both the patient and the dentist to seal the moving soft tissue. This enables precise capture of these areas during the final impression taking. The aim of our novel approach was to incorporate a temperature sensitive rim into the tray design of the printed individual impression tray.

Based on an intraoral scan, an individual impression tray (Figure 4) was designed using CAD software (inLab, Dentsply Sirona, Charlotte, NC, USA). This was achieved by setting an insertion direction, blocking out undercuts, defining the length of the tray rim, and digitally positioning the tray handle.

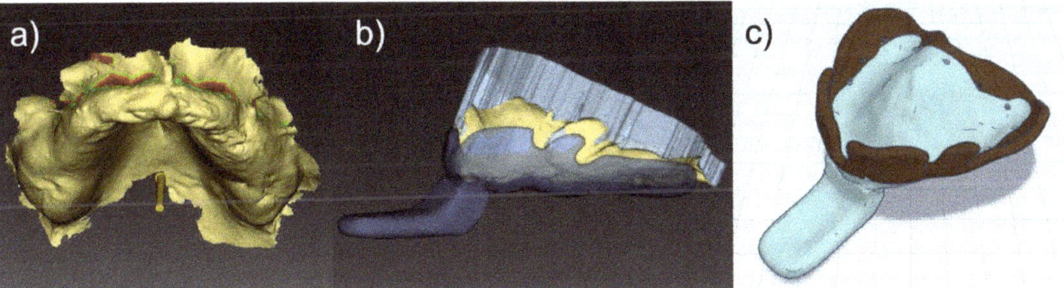

Figure 4. Design of a dual-material customized impression tray. (**a**) intraoral scan with undercuts shown in red, (**b**) finished one-piece custom tray design, (**c**) thermoplastic compound material (brown), and rigid (cyan) parts separated into two STL files.

Subsequently, using additional software (Tinkercad, Autodesk, San Rafael, CA, USA), the resulting STL was split into two parts. Hereby, the cut was drawn along the occlusal plane, separating around 1.5 cm of the part touching the vestibulum from the central tray-body. Using a multi-material printer equipped with an independent dual extrusion (IDEX) system (Sigmax R19, BCN3D, Barcelona, Spain) allowed for combining two materials with different properties into one print. This creates the possibility of using a rigid material for the tray body, whereas the part which comes in contact with the mobile mucosa was printed using a temperature-sensitive material (Figure 5).

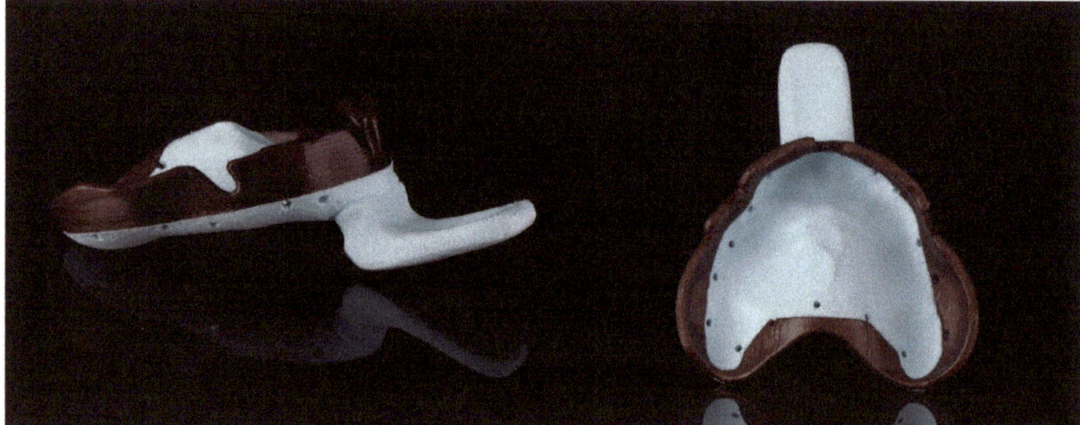

Figure 5. Dual material customized impression tray. The rigid body was manufactured with a polyethylene terephthalate glycol (PETG) filament (Trayfill), the rim was printed with a thermoplastic filament.

Compared to the conventional approach, our dual material design with an integrated functional margin allows for a clean and fast workflow, a reduced treatment time, and, thus, increased patient comfort. However, until there are software enhancements that fully automatize the dual-material custom design process, this production workflow must be considered time-consuming and therefore may not yet be cost-effective.

3.3. Surgical Guides

The manufacturing of surgical guides with FFF can offer a simple and cost-effective workflow. Inexpensive, biodegradable, and steam-sterilizable filaments [30] are an interesting choice of materials. In a former evaluation of the manufacturing procedure of surgical guides, difficulties regarding precision and the fitting of FFF printed surgical guides on a cast model were observed [31]. In contrast, other studies showed no difference when compared with surgical guides produced by means of DLP [32]. Besides accuracy, other factors resulted in a deviation between the planned and realized implant positions of >1 mm [33,34].

A workflow has been established in which surgical guides are planned digitally and manufactured using FFF. Two different design softwares were used (CoDiagnostix, Dental Wings GmbH, Chemnitz, Germany; ImplantStudio, 3Shape, Copenhagen, Denmark). In both cases, the exported STL file was transferred to the slicer software (PrusaSlicer, Prusa, Prague, Czech Republic) and printed without further modification (Figure 6a). A Prusa mini+ printer (Prusa, Prague, Czech Republic) with a biodegradable filament (Greentec Pro, Extrudr FD3D GmbH, Lauterach, Austria) was used for additive manufacturing. Although medical approval for this filament has yet to be obtained, pending cytotoxicity tests show promising initial results. The detailed view of the guiding structure of the coDiagnostic surgical guide (Figure 6b) reveals a smooth and precise surface, nevertheless, the individual layers of the FFF manufacturing process are visible.

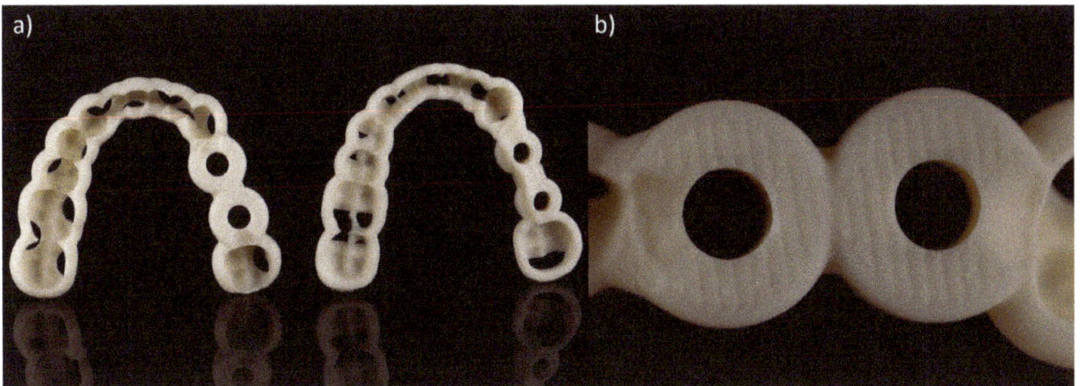

Figure 6. (**a**) Two FFF printed implant templates planed with coDiagnostix (l.) and ImplantStudio (r.). In both cases, the exported STL file was transferred to the slicer software and printed without further modification. (**b**) Close-up of the coDiagnostix surgical guide showing the guiding structure. The individual layers of the filament print become visible.

The accuracy of surgical guides manufactured with FFF is a discussed topic since FFF is considered less precise than SLA/DLP. The in vitro accuracy of placed implants in relation to their virtual position with guides printed with FFF has already been investigated. Implants inserted using FFF printed guides showed equivalent deviations to those inserted using SLA guides and were within clinical tolerances of <1 mm [30]. It was shown that printed drill sleeves integrated into the surgical guide do not cause more deviation in the implant position, compared to traditional metal sleeves. This can be a major advantage in clinical applications, especially considering the potentially good biocompatibility of the biodegradable filaments.

Great potential lies in the simplicity of handling and accessibility of the manufacturing process. The easy operability of the CAM software allows even first-time users to achieve useable objects. The surgical guides and the support structure are removable without tools. Without further post-processing, the guides can be steam-sterilized and directly used. Furthermore, this production route offers cost-effective manufacturing of surgical guides using FFF with printers available at competitive prices, software available free of charge, and a material cost of 50 cents per surgical guide. If a sleeveless design is adopted, further cost savings can be achieved. Further research on the design and optimization of surgical guides, as well as studies on the clinical application, are required. The influence of metal debris of the sleeves compromising the implant bed in conventional surgical guides compared to filament residues in sleeveless applications needs to be investigated.

4. Conclusions and Future Perspectives

Non-load bearing applications are a potential field of use for FFF in dentistry. Models, trays, and prototypes for denture try-ins can be manufactured with FFF. Materials which are certified are commercially accessible or under investigation. Multi-material printers are available which allow the easy testing of innovative concepts for the use of FFF in dentistry. The inexpensive initial cost of the printer and the price of materials allow FFF to be competitive. The possibility of open printers that allow the use of third-party materials seems to be a huge benefit. In most cases, the productivity of FFF printers is inferior compared to DLP systems. However, high productivity and high quantity do not always consider the needs of smaller medical clinics where printer capacity cannot always be fully utilized.

Author Contributions: Conceptualization, J.L.; F.B.; J.N. and B.C.S.; methodology, J.L.; F.B.; B.C.S.; formal analysis, J.L.; G.W.; investigation, J.L.; F.B.; J.N.; S.R.; resources, S.W.; data curation, S.W.; C.W.; S.P.; writing—original draft preparation, J.L.; F.B. and J.N.; writing—review and editing, J.L.; F.B.; J.N. and B.C.S.; visualization, G.W. and S.R.; supervision, B.C.S. All authors have read and agreed to the published version of the manuscript.

Funding: The article processing charge was funded by the Baden-Wuerttemberg Ministry of Science, Research and Art and the University of Freiburg in the funding programme Open Access Publishing.

Informed Consent Statement: Written informed consent has been obtained from the patient(s) to publish this paper.

Conflicts of Interest: The authors declare no conflict of interest.

References

1. Goodacre, B.J.; Goodacre, C.J.; Baba, N.Z.; Kattadiyil, M.T. Comparison of denture base adaptation between CAD-CAM and conventional fabrication techniques. *J. Prosthet. Dent.* **2016**, *116*, 249–256. [CrossRef] [PubMed]
2. Romanyk, D.L.; Martinez, Y.T.; Veldhuis, S.; Rae, N.; Guo, Y.; Sirovica, S.; Fleming, G.J.P.; Addison, O. Strength-limiting damage in lithium silicate glass-ceramics associated with CAD–CAM. *Dent. Mater.* **2019**, *35*, 98–104. [CrossRef] [PubMed]
3. ASTM. ISO/ASTM 52900. In *Additive Manufacturing—General Principles—Terminology*; Beuth: Berlin, Germany, 2018; p. 73.
4. Revilla-León, M.; Özcan, M. Additive Manufacturing Technologies Used for Processing Polymers: Current Status and Potential Application in Prosthetic Dentistry. *J. Prosthodont.* **2019**, *28*, 146–158. [CrossRef] [PubMed]
5. Schweiger, J.; Edelhoff, D.; Güth, J.-F. 3D Printing in Digital Prosthetic Dentistry: An Overview of Recent Developments in Additive Manufacturing. *J. Clin. Med.* **2021**, *10*, 2010. [CrossRef] [PubMed]
6. Hull, C.W. Apparatus for Production of Three-Dimensional Objects by Stereolithography. U.S. Patent 4,575,330, 8 August 1984.
7. Zguris, Z. How Mechanical Properties of Stereolithography 3D Prints are affected by UV Curing, Formlabs White Paper. Available online: https://3d.formlabs.com/mechanical-properties-of-uv-cured-3d-prints/ (accessed on 26 May 2021).
8. Formlabs. White Paper 3d Printing Custom Trays. Available online: https://3d.formlabs.com/white-paper-de-3d-printing-custom-trays/ (accessed on 31 May 2021).
9. Crump, S.S. Apparatus and Method for Creating Three-Dimensional Objects. U.S. Patent 5,121,329, 5 September 1989.
10. Comb, J.; Priedman, W.; Turley, P.W. FDM Technology Process Improvements. In Proceedings of the 1994 International Solid Freeform Fabrication Symposium, Austin, TX, USA, 8–10 August 1994.
11. Ligon, S.C.; Liska, R.; Stampfl, J.; Gurr, M.; Mülhaupt, R. Polymers for 3D Printing and Customized Additive Manufacturing. *Chem. Rev.* **2017**, *117*, 10212–10290. [CrossRef] [PubMed]
12. Stratasys. Thermoplastic: The Strongest Choise for 3D Printing, FDM Thermoplastic 3d Printing White Paper. Available online: https://www.stratasys.com/explore/whitepaper/thermoplastics (accessed on 26 May 2021).
13. Solvay. Radel® PPSU HC AM Filament NT1. Available online: https://www.solvayamshop.com/ccrz__ProductDetails?viewState=DetailView&cartID=&sku=Z58-40004&portalUser=&store=&cclcl=en_US (accessed on 26 May 2021).
14. FibreTuff. Fibre Tuff II Data Sheet. Available online: https://img1.wsimg.com/blobby/go/4fc374e5-752e-4d9c-9806-458efb923e97/downloads/FibreTuff%20II%20Data%20Sheet.pdf?ver=1621429055001 (accessed on 26 May 2021).
15. Solvay. KetaSpire® PEEK HC FILAMENT CF10 LS1. Available online: https://www.solvayamshop.com/ccrz__ProductDetails?viewState=DetailView&cartID=&sku=Z58-40002&portalUser=&store=&cclcl=en_US (accessed on 26 May 2021).
16. Honigmann, P.; Sharma, N.; Okolo, B.; Popp, U.; Msallem, B.; Thieringer, F.M. Patient-Specific Surgical Implants Made of 3D Printed PEEK: Material, Technology, and Scope of Surgical Application. *BioMed Res. Int.* **2018**, *2018*, 4520636. [CrossRef] [PubMed]
17. Sharma, N.; Honigmann, P.; Cao, S.; Thieringer, F. Dimensional characteristics of FDM 3D printed PEEK implant for craniofacial reconstructions. *Trans. Addit. Manuf. Meets Med.* **2020**, *2*. [CrossRef]
18. Han, X.; Sharma, N.; Xu, Z.; Scheideler, L.; Geis-Gerstorfer, J.; Rupp, F.; Thieringer, F.M.; Spintzyk, S. An In Vitro Study of Osteoblast Response on Fused-Filament Fabrication 3D Printed PEEK for Dental and Cranio-Maxillofacial Implants. *J. Clin. Med.* **2019**, *8*, 771. [CrossRef] [PubMed]
19. JohannesWeithasGmbH. Arfona Impression Tray Filament. Available online: https://www.weithas.de/de/prothetik/3d_druck_dental/fdm_3d-druck_loeffel_dental_filament (accessed on 26 May 2021).
20. AdvancedBiomedicalTechnology. MeDFila® 3D Printing Filament. Available online: https://advbiomedtech.com/medfila/ (accessed on 26 May 2021).
21. Kim, S.-Y.; Shin, Y.-S.; Jung, H.-D.; Hwang, C.-J.; Baik, H.-S.; Cha, J.-Y. Precision and trueness of dental models manufactured with different 3-dimensional printing techniques. *Am. J. Orthod. Dentofac. Orthop.* **2018**, *153*, 144–153. [CrossRef] [PubMed]
22. Etemad-Shahidi, Y.; Qallandar, O.B.; Evenden, J.; Alifui-Segbaya, F.; Ahmed, K.E. Accuracy of 3-Dimensionally Printed Full-Arch Dental Models: A Systematic Review. *J. Clin. Med.* **2020**, *9*, 3357. [CrossRef] [PubMed]
23. 3dk.berlin. Filadental Gips Weiß. Available online: https://3dk.berlin/de/filadental/502-filadental-gips-weiss-4251163216986.html (accessed on 31 May 2021).

24. JohannesWeithasGmbH. Weiton-3D Gips Bio-Filament. Available online: https://www.weithas.de/de/prothetik/3d_druck_dental/dentalgips_bio_filament (accessed on 31 May 2021).
25. Chen, H.; Yang, X.; Chen, L.; Wang, Y.; Sun, Y. Application of FDM three-dimensional printing technology in the digital manufacture of custom edentulous mandible trays. *Sci. Rep.* **2016**, *6*, 19207. [CrossRef] [PubMed]
26. Sun, Y.; Chen, H.; Li, H.; Deng, K.; Zhao, T.; Wang, Y.; Zhou, Y. Clinical evaluation of final impressions from three-dimensional printed custom trays. *Sci. Rep.* **2017**, *7*, 14958. [CrossRef] [PubMed]
27. IGO3D. Dental 3D Agency Trayfill Filament. Available online: https://www.igo3d.com/dental-3d-agency-trayfill-filament (accessed on 31 May 2021).
28. Arcuri, L.; Lorenzi, C.; Vanni, A.; Bianchi, N.; Dolci, A.; Arcuri, C. Comparison of the accuracy of intraoral scanning and conventional impression techniques on implants: A review. *J. Biol. Regul. Homeost. Agents* **2020**, *34*, 89–97. [PubMed]
29. Ender, A.; Zimmermann, M.; Mehl, A. Accuracy of complete- and partial-arch impressions of actual intraoral scanning systems in vitro. *Int. J. Comput. Dent.* **2019**, *22*, 11–19. [PubMed]
30. Pieralli, S.; Spies, B.C.; Hromadnik, V.; Nicic, R.; Beuer, F.; Wesemann, C. How Accurate Is Oral Implant Installation Using Surgical Guides Printed from a Degradable and Steam-Sterilized Biopolymer? *J. Clin. Med.* **2020**, *9*, 2322. [CrossRef] [PubMed]
31. Sommacal, B.; Savic, M.; Filippi, A.; Kühl, S.; Thieringer, F.M. Evaluation of Two 3D Printers for Guided Implant Surgery. *Int. J. Oral Maxillofac. Implants* **2018**, *33*, 743–746. [CrossRef] [PubMed]
32. Sun, Y.; Ding, Q.; Tang, L.; Zhang, L.; Sun, Y.; Xie, Q. Accuracy of a chairside fused deposition modeling 3D-printed single-tooth surgical template for implant placement: An in vitro comparison with a light cured template. *J. Cranio-Maxillofac. Surg.* **2019**, *47*, 1216–1221. [CrossRef] [PubMed]
33. Zhou, W.; Liu, Z.; Song, L.; Kuo, C.-l.; Shafer, D.M. Clinical Factors Affecting the Accuracy of Guided Implant Surgery—A Systematic Review and Meta-analysis. *J. Evid. Based Dent. Pract.* **2018**, *18*, 28–40. [CrossRef] [PubMed]
34. Bover-Ramos, F.; Viña-Almunia, J.; Cervera-Ballester, J.; Peñarrocha-Diago, M.; García-Mira, B. Accuracy of Implant Placement with Computer-Guided Surgery: A Systematic Review and Meta-Analysis Comparing Cadaver, Clinical, and In Vitro Studies. *Int. J. Oral Maxillofac. Implants* **2018**, *33*, 101–115. [CrossRef] [PubMed]

applied
sciences

MDPI

Article

Effect of Printing Layer Thickness on the Trueness and Margin Quality of 3D-Printed Interim Dental Crowns

Gülce Çakmak [1], Alfonso Rodriguez Cuellar [2], Mustafa Borga Donmez [3], Martin Schimmel [1,4], Samir Abou-Ayash [1,*], Wei-En Lu [5] and Burak Yilmaz [1,6,7]

[1]   Department of Reconstructive Dentistry and Gerodontology, School of Dental Medicine, University of Bern, 3010 Bern, Switzerland; guelce.cakmak@zmk.unibe.ch (G.Ç.); martin.schimmel@zmk.unibe.ch (M.S.); burak.yilmaz@zmk.unibe.ch (B.Y.)
[2]   Department of Periodontology, Clinica Dental Rodriguez Dental Clinic, Mexico City 03100, Mexico; alfonso_rodriguez@my.unitec.edu.mx
[3]   Department of Prosthodontics, Biruni University Faculty of Dentistry, 34010 Istanbul, Turkey; bdonmez@biruni.edu.tr
[4]   Division of Gerodontology and Removable Prosthodontics, University Clinics of Dental Medicine, University of Geneva, 1205 Geneva, Switzerland
[5]   Division of Biostatistics, The Ohio State University College of Public Health, Columbus, OH 43210, USA; lu.1408@buckeyemail.osu.edu
[6]   Department of Restorative, Preventive and Pediatric Dentistry, School of Dental Medicine, University of Bern, 3010 Bern, Switzerland
[7]   Division of Restorative and Prosthetic Dentistry, The Ohio State University College of Dentistry, Columbus, OH 43210, USA
*   Correspondence: samir.abou-ayash@zmk.unibe.ch; Tel.: +41-(0)31-632-8705

Citation: Çakmak, G.; Cuellar, A.R.; Donmez, M.B.; Schimmel, M.; Abou-Ayash, S.; Lu, W.-E.; Yilmaz, B. Effect of Printing Layer Thickness on the Trueness and Margin Quality of 3D-Printed Interim Dental Crowns. *Appl. Sci.* **2021**, *11*, 9246. https://doi.org/10.3390/app11199246

Academic Editor: Kathrin Becker

Received: 8 September 2021
Accepted: 2 October 2021
Published: 5 October 2021

Abstract: The information in the literature on the effect of printing layer thickness on interim 3D-printed crowns is limited. In the present study, the effect of layer thickness on the trueness and margin quality of 3D-printed composite resin crowns was investigated and compared with milled crowns. The crowns were printed in 3 different layer thicknesses (20, 50, and 100 μm) by using a hybrid resin based on acrylic esters with inorganic microfillers or milled from polymethylmethacrylate (PMMA) discs and digitized with an intraoral scanner (test scans). The compare tool of the 3D analysis software was used to superimpose the test scans and the computer-aided design file by using the manual alignment tool and to virtually separate the surfaces. Deviations at different surfaces on crowns were calculated by using root mean square (RMS). Margin quality of crowns was examined under a stereomicroscope and graded. The data were evaluated with one-way ANOVA and Tukey HSD tests. The layer thickness affected the trueness and margin quality of 3D-printed interim crowns. Milled crowns had higher trueness on intaglio and intaglio occlusal surfaces than 100 μm-layer thickness crowns. Milled crowns had the highest margin quality, while 20 μm and 100 μm layer thickness printed crowns had the lowest. The quality varied depending on the location of the margin.

Keywords: 3D printing; additive manufacturing; interim crowns; provisional crowns; trueness; accuracy; layer thickness; margin quality

1. Introduction

The introduction of digital technologies into dental practice has facilitated manufacturing, as computer aided design-computer aided manufacturing (CAD-CAM) enabled the fabrication of accurate definitive restorations [1]. CAD-CAM manufacturing can be subtractive (milling) [2] or additive, and the interest has recently shifted towards additive manufacturing technologies that are also known as rapid prototyping or 3-dimensional (3D) printing [3–5].

3D-printing manufactures an object by building up consecutive layers [5,6] and is used for a wide range of dental applications including diagnostic and master models, surgical guides, complete dentures, occlusal splints, impression trays, implants, metal crowns, copings, and frameworks [4,7–13]. Printing has certain advantages over milling as less waste material is produced, multiple products with more complex geometries can be fabricated, and less energy is consumed [14,15]. Moreover, due to an increased accuracy and speed, of 3D-printing has increased its popularity in the dental field [16]. Several different 3D-printing technologies, namely stereolithography (SLA), digital light processing (DLP), material jetting (MJ), material extrusion (ME), binder jetting, powder bed fusion (PBF), sheet lamination, and direct energy deposition, are currently available for polymers [7]. However, among these technologies, the popularity of DLP, which is based on the UV light activation of the photosensitive resin [17], is increasing for the fabrication of dental prosthesis [4,18].

Interim restorations are an essential component of the prosthodontic treatment as they act as a prototype of the definitive prosthesis providing esthetics, pulp protection, tooth positional stability, and soft tissue management [19,20]. Conventional interim restorations are fabricated commonly by using polymethylmethacrylate (PMMA) due to its accessibility, ease of fabrication and repair, low cost, biocompatibility, and stability in the oral environment [19–21]. Even though direct fabrication of acrylic resin interim crowns is feasible [22], polymerization shrinkage, possible biologic reactions due to the residual monomers, and marginal and occlusal discrepancies can be observed [20,22,23]. The indirect fabrication of these restorations with CAD-CAM technologies led to a better internal fit [20] and marginal integrity [24], enabling successful and long-lasting restorations [20]. Both subtractive manufacturing and 3D-printing technologies are applicable for the fabrication of interim restorations [19].

Efficiency of 3D-printing is affected by the layer thickness, laser intensity, laser speed, build angle, the geometry of the supporting structures, and printing technology [14,21,25–27]. Layer thickness is a controllable parameter that affects the accuracy, which is defined by trueness and precision [28], of the final restoration [7]. Therefore, setting the appropriate layer thickness is crucial to achieve optimum results. In addition, layer thickness was shown to affect the printing speed and printing accuracy [16]. In general, the layer thickness of a 3D-printer based on photopolymerization ranges between 20 to 150 μm [7].

Previous studies on 3D-printed interim materials have mainly focused on the effect of printing orientation [14,18,25,26,29], while the effect of layer thickness was assessed primarily when 3D-printed dental models [16], trial dentures [30], and custom trays [13] were printed. Only one study investigated the effect of printing orientation and layer thickness on the fit of 3-unit implant-supported fixed partial dentures [31]. To the authors' knowledge, no study has evaluated the effect of layer thickness on the accuracy of 3D-printed interim crowns. Therefore, the aim of this study was to investigate the trueness and margin quality of interim crowns printed in 3 different layer thicknesses (20, 50, and 100 μm) comparing with that of milled PMMA crowns. The null hypotheses were that (i) fabrication technique would not affect the trueness of the crowns and (ii) fabrication technique and margin location would not affect the margin quality of the restorations.

2. Materials and Methods

2.1. Model and Crown Data Acquisition

A mandibular right first molar tooth in a dentate typodont model (ANA-4, Frasaco GmbH, Tettnang, Germany) was prepared with a 1-mm-wide chamfer finish line to simulate a complete coverage crown preparation. The maxillary and mandibular typodont models and both models when in occlusion were scanned by using an intraoral scanner (Medit i500 v. 1.2.1, Medit, Seoul, Korea) that has a precision of 25 μm, according to the manufacturers' recommended scan strategy. The scans were converted to standard tessellation language (STL) files (Figure 1). A complete-coverage restoration was designed to simulate an interim crown by using a dental design software program (Exocad Dental CAD2.2, Exocad GmbH, Darmstadt, Germany) with 30 μm cement space gap [26]. This design was saved as the reference scan STL file (RS-STL), which was then used to fabricate 3D-printed ($n = 30$) and milled (control) ($n = 10$) molar crowns.

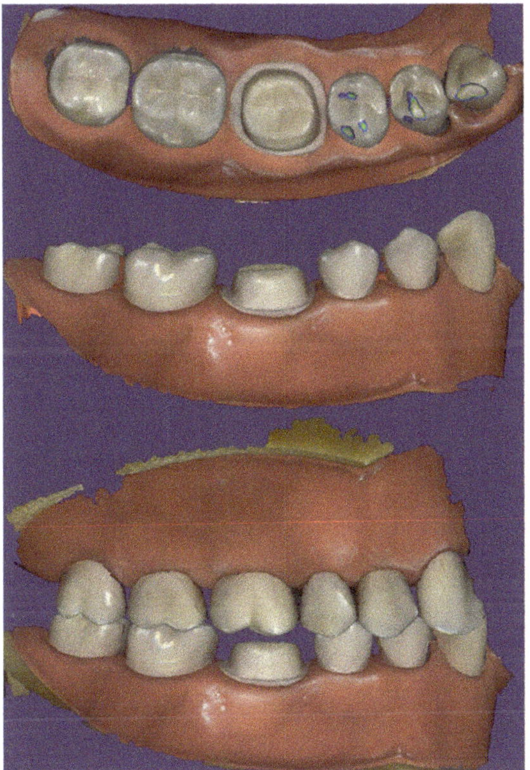

Figure 1. Mandibular right first molar preparation.

2.2. Crown Fabrication

Three different layer thicknesses (20 µm, 50 µm, and 100 µm) were used to print the crowns ($n = 10$ per layer thickness). First, the RS-STL file of the crown was imported to DLP software (MoonRay S100, SprintRay Inc, Los Angeles, CA, USA) to arrange the build angle and support configuration. As recommended by the manufacturer of the printing resin material (Nextdent Crown and Bridge Micro Filled Hybrid-MFH, C&B; 3D systems, Soesterberg, The Netherlands), the occlusal surface of the crown was angled 45° from the print area for improved occlusal surface details. The semiautomatically created support structures were checked and supports that were automatically created on the margin area and fitting surfaces of the crowns were manually eliminated. Then, this configuration was duplicated 10 times and 10 identical crown configurations were arranged in the build platform of the DLP printer (MoonRay S100 Software, SprintRay Inc, Los Angeles, CA, USA) to print all crowns in the same configuration. This configuration was further saved for 3 different layer thicknesses to print the crowns in identical configuration, but by using different layer thicknesses. The crowns were printed with the DLP printer (MoonRay S100, SprintRay Inc, Los Angeles, CA, USA) and an interim printing resin material (N1 shade, Nextdent Crown and Bridge Micro Filled Hybrid-MFH, C&B; 3D systems, Soesterberg, The Netherlands, Lot: XH312N21) by using 20 µm, 50 µm, or 100 µm ($n = 10$) layer thickness. According to the manufacturer, the printing material has 100–130 MPa flexural strength, 2400–2600 MPa flexural modulus, $\leq$70 µg/mm^3 sorption, and $\leq$15.5 µg/mm^3 solubility.

The DLP printer has UV DLP projector, LED-based light source, and 405 nm blue-violet light resin curing unit. After printing, the printed crowns were removed from the platform by using a putty knife, ultrasonically rinsed for 5 min (first 3 min then 2 min) in 96% clean alcohol solution (Alcohol isopropilico, Quimi Klean, Mexico City, Mexico) according to the manufacturers' recommendations. After ensuring that the crowns were dry and free of alcohol residue, they were postpolymerized by using an ultraviolet polymerizing unit (SprintRay Procure Model SRP1811A, SprintRay Inc, Los Angeles, CA, USA) (405 nm LED arrays) for 30 min (Figure 2).

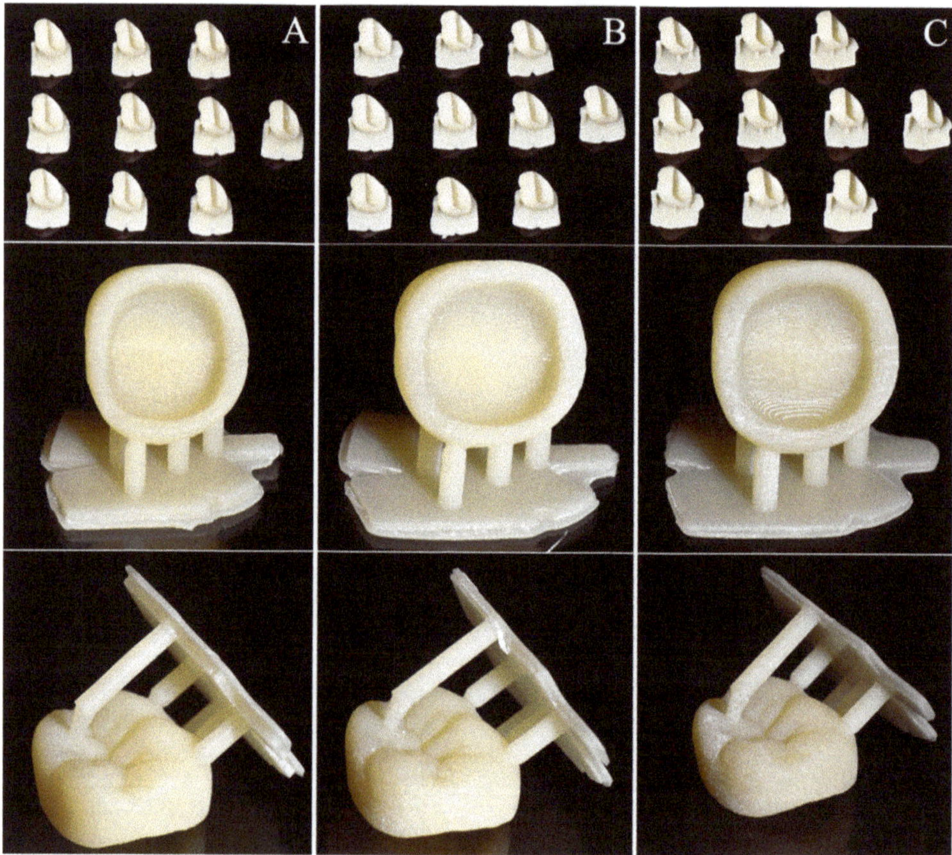

Figure 2. 3D-printed interim crowns ((**A**): 20 μm crowns; (**B**): 50 μm crowns; (**C**): 100 μm crowns).

The support structures were cut and trimmed after cooling and the surface was gently smoothened to prevent errors during the alignment procedure.

In the milling technique, crowns were milled (Wieland Zenotec mini, V6.12.04, Wieland Dental + Technik GmbH & Co.KG, Pforzheim, Germany) from a polymethyl methacrylate (PMMA) block (A2 shade, Lot number: HL201104, Upcera, Shenzhen Upcera Dental Technology Co. Ltd., Shenzen, Guandong, China). The designed STL file was inserted in the block to mill 10 identical crowns. The support structures were cut and trimmed after milling, and the support surfaces were gently smoothened. All crown fabrication processes were performed by one operator (G. Ç).

2.3. Crown Analysis

All crowns were examined under optical magnification loupe (3.5×) to ensure that they were free from any defects and no adjustments were made on the inner surfaces of the crowns [26]. Crowns were then kept in dry and lightproof boxes to scan within 48 h after the fabrication. First, the scanner was calibrated and then the printed and milled crowns were scanned by using an intraoral scanner (Medit i500 v. 1.2.1, Medit, Seoul, Korea) by the same operator (G. Ç) and the scan files were converted to STL files (test-scan STL). During the scan, the crowns were hold with small tweezers and as the intraoral scanner utilized has a filter for colors, the parts in contact with the tweezers were scanned afterwards.

For the deviation analysis, root mean square (RMS) was used to indicate how far the deviations were from zero between the 2 different datasets [32]. A low RMS value indicated a high degree of 3D matching of the superimposed data, which translated to high trueness [33]. First, test-scan STL files and designed crown STL file (RS-STL) were imported into a software (Medit Link, Medit, Seoul, Korea). Compare tool (Medit Compare v1.1.1.61, Medit, Seoul, Korea) of the software, which has an automatic alignment tool was used for the superimposition, virtually separation of the surfaces, and RMS calculation. For the superimposition, RS-STL was moved to the reference data and test-scan STL was moved to the target data by using the alignment tool of the software. Then, manual alignment tool of the software was selected and 3 reference points; central fossa, mesial and distal triangular fossae were selected both in the reference and target data. Test-scan STL files were then superimposed over the RS-STL file (Figure 3).

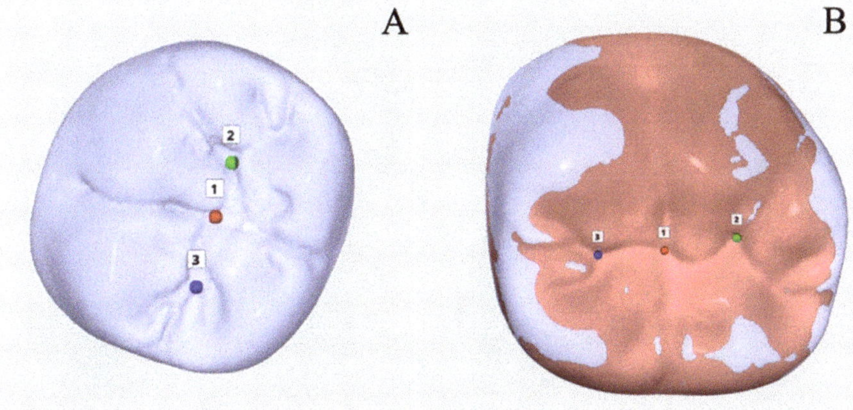

Figure 3. (**A**): Reference points determined for the superimposition of STL files (1: Central fossa; 2: Distal triangular fossa; 3: Mesial triangular fossa), (**B**): Superimposition of the Test-scan STL over the RS-STL by using these points.

To generate color maps to represent the 3D deviation, deviation display mode of the software was used. The maximum/minimum critical (nominal) values were set at +50/−50 µm with a tolerance range of +10/−10 µm, respectively [34]. After the superimposition, color-difference maps were created to compare the test scan STL file and the RS-STL for the overall RMS, which includes all surfaces of the crowns. The software automatically calculated the RMS from the color-difference maps, without the need for an additional formula. For the RMS of external, intaglio, marginal area, and intaglio occlusal surfaces of the crowns, the test-scan STL files and the RS-STL file were imported again, and these surfaces were virtually separated both in test-scan STL files and RS-STL file [34] dividing crowns into 4 different parts by using the edit mode of the software. After separation, the superimposition was done once again for each surface (external, intaglio, marginal area, and intaglio occlusal surfaces) of each crown by using automatic alignment mode of the software, and the color-difference maps were generated for those surfaces and the RMS values were automatically calculated (Figure 4). The areas with deviations exceeding the scale utilized were presented as gray by the software. However, all areas were included in the RMS calculation.

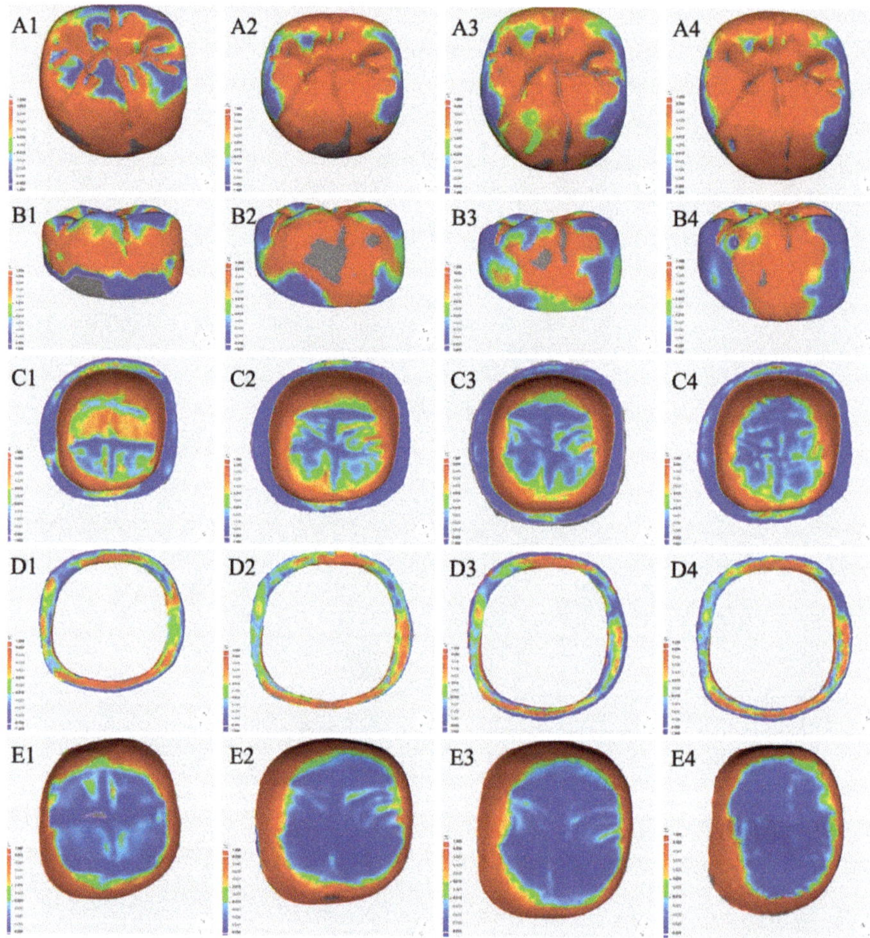

Figure 4. Color maps generated by the superimposition of the milled (**1**), 20 µm (**2**), 50 µm (**3**), and 100 µm (**4**) crown meshes over reference data ((**A**): Overall RMS; (**B**): External RMS; (**C**): Internal RMS; (**D**): Marginal RMS; (**E**): Intaglio Occlusal RMS).

For margin quality comparison, each crown was randomly numbered by an independent individual, and then visually examined with an optical microscope (Zeiss) under ×60 magnification by a single operator (G.Ç.) who was blinded about the numbering, and a grading system from 1 to 3 was used as performed in a previous study [29]. Grade 1 crown margins indicated rough edges similar to layers. Grade 2 crown margins indicated slightly rough edges similar to waves. Grade 3 crown margins indicated smooth edges (Figure 5). Margin quality was examined at each margin location (buccal, lingual, mesial, and distal) of each crown, and the average was calculated for each printed or milled crown.

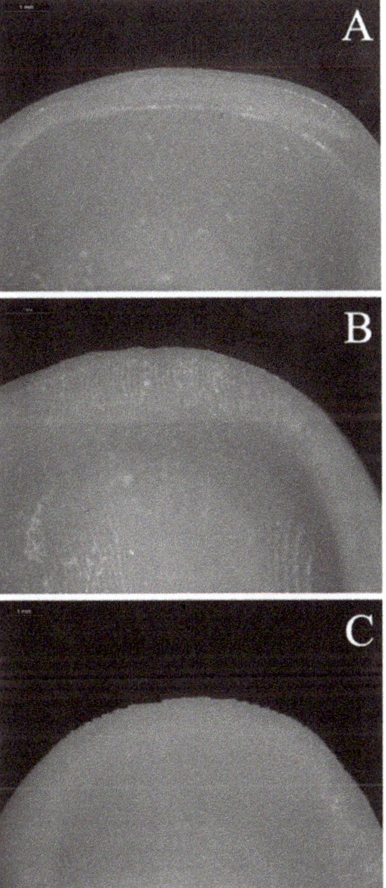

Figure 5. Margins according to the grading system ((**A**): Grade 3; (**B**): Grade 2; (**C**): Grade 1).

2.4. Statistical Analysis

The statistical evaluation of the data was performed by using the statistical software R. Normality assumption was verified using the Shapiro Wilks test. Difference in RMS values between fabrication technique within each area of measurement, difference in average quality rating between fabrication technique, and difference in quality rating between margin location for each fabrication technique was analyzed by using the one-way analysis of variance (ANOVA). Additionally, pairwise comparisons within the groups were analyzed with Tukey HSD Post-Hoc analysis ($\alpha = 0.05$).

3. Results

One-way ANOVA results of the RMS values of each surface are presented in Table 1, and Figure 6 illustrates the RMS at each measured surface for control and different layer-thickness groups.

Table 1. Mean RMS (µm) values ± standard deviations for milled and 3D-printed interim crowns. Different superscript lowercase letters in same column indicate significant differences among groups ($p < 0.05$).

Layer Thickness	Overall RMS (µm)	External RMS (µm)	Intaglio RMS (µm)	Marginal RMS (µm)	Intaglio Occlusal RMS (µm)
Control (Milled)	64.5 ±10.94 [a]	54 ±21.29 [a]	32.6 ±15.01 [a]	11.3 ±14.36 [a]	31.5 ±6.92 [a]
20 µm	56.1 ±10.7 [a]	59.4 ±10.7 [a]	49.9 ±12.13 [ab]	14.9 ±9.57 [a]	33.4 ± 2.22 [ab]
50 µm	53.3 ±9.3 [a]	48.5 ±13.67 [a]	45.4 ±15.75 [ab]	9.1 ±8.02 [a]	34.7 ±1.83 [ab]
100 µm	61.3 ±15.31 [a]	62.4 ±18.21 [a]	52.8 ±17.32 [b]	14.6 ±9.94 [a]	41.5 ±12.55 [b]
p values	0.145	0.263	0.026	0.576	0.024

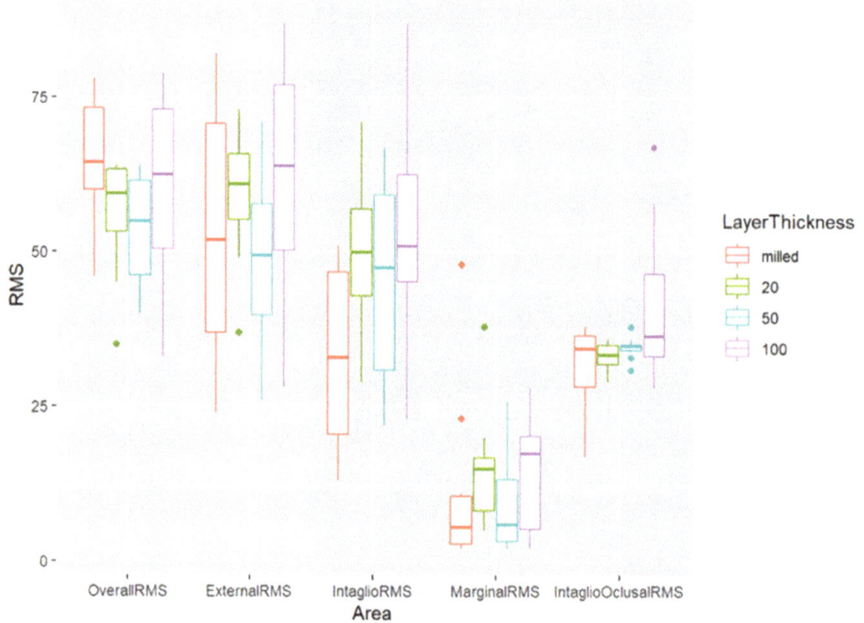

Figure 6. Box-plot graph of the RMS values of milled and 3D-printed interim crowns according to different surfaces.

Significant differences were observed among fabrication techniques for intaglio and intaglio occlusal surface RMS values ($p \leq 0.026$). Milled crowns presented significantly lower RMS values than 100 µm crowns at both intaglio ($p = 0.025$, estimated difference in means: −20.2 µm) and intaglio occlusal ($p = 0.021$, estimated difference in means: −10 µm) surfaces. Every other pairwise comparison for intaglio ($p \geq 0.251$) and intaglio occlusal ($p \geq 0.178$) surfaces were nonsignificant.

Average margin quality of the crowns showed significant differences (Figure 7); based on the 3-point scale, milled crowns presented higher quality than the others ($p < 0.001$ vs. 20 µm, estimated difference in means: 1.25 points; $p = 0.001$ vs. 50 µm, estimated difference in means: 0.68 points; and $p < 0.001$ vs. 100 µm, estimated difference in means: 1.53 points).

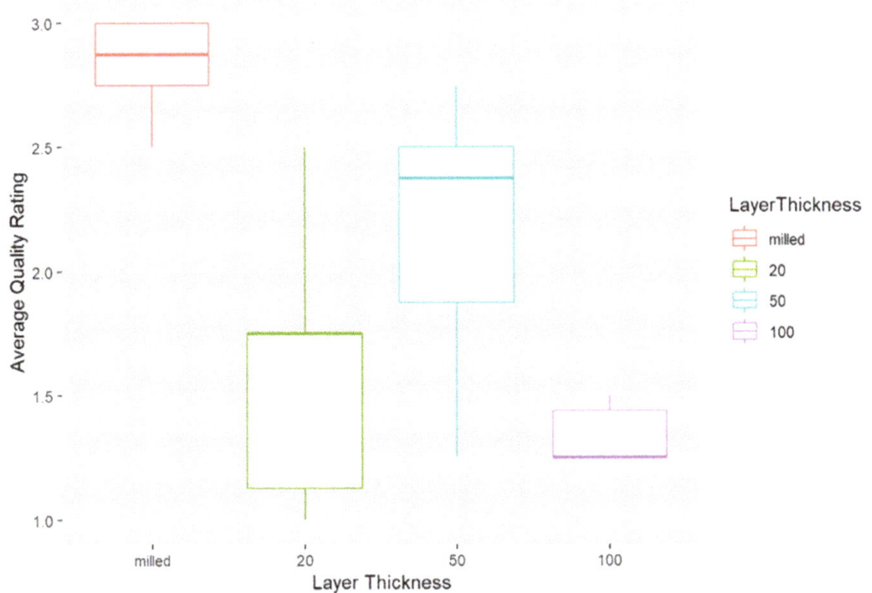

Figure 7. Average margin quality of all groups, evaluated by using a 3-point scale, ranging from 1 (worst marginal quality) to 3 (best marginal quality).

The margin quality of 50 µm crowns was higher than that of 20 µm ($p = 0.006$, estimated difference in means: 0.58 points) and 100 µm ($p < 0.001$, estimated difference in means: 0.85 points) crowns. The difference between 20 µm crowns and 100 µm crowns was nonsignificant ($p = 0.348$). Table 2 summarizes the p values when the Tukey HSD test was applied to analyze the effect of margin location on the margin quality within each fabrication technique.

Table 2. p values for the pairwise comparison between different margin locations for milled and 3D-printed interim crowns. $p < 0.05$ indicate significant differences between locations.

	Locations					
Layer Thickness	**Buccal-Lingual**	**Buccal-Mesial**	**Buccal-Distal**	**Lingual-Mesial**	**Lingual-Distal**	**Mesial-Distal**
Control (Milled)	0.005	0.03	0.005	0.885	>0.05	0.885
20 µm	0.121	0.762	0.988	0.566	0.223	0.914
50 µm	0.765	0.765	0.988	>0.05	0.915	0.915
100 µm	<0.001	0.831	0.831	<0.001	<0.001	>0.05

No significant differences were found between the quality of the margins at different locations for 20 µm ($p \geq 0.121$) and 50 µm ($p \geq 0.765$) crowns. However, margin quality of milled ($p = 0.002$) and 100 µm ($p < 0.001$) crowns were significantly affected by the margin location. The mesial, distal, and lingual margin quality of the milled crowns was similar ($p \geq 0.885$), while buccal margin quality was inferior to that at other locations ($p \leq 0.03$). For the 100 µm crowns, lingual margin quality was higher compared with other locations ($p < 0.001$); the differences among other locations were nonsignificant ($p \geq 0.831$). The margin quality in control and each layer thickness groups according to the margin location is presented in Figure 8.

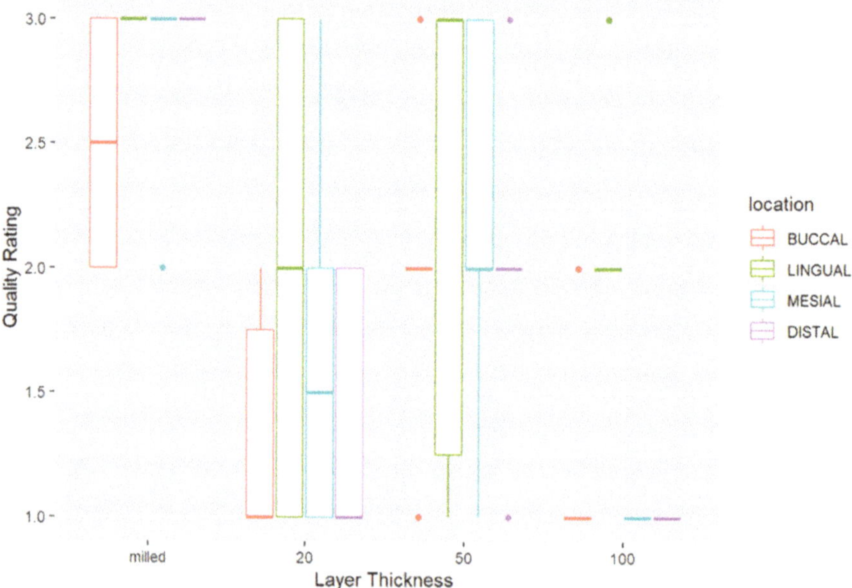

Figure 8. Margin quality of groups according to margin location, evaluated by using a 3-point scale that ranged from 1 (worst marginal quality) to 3 (best marginal quality).

4. Discussion

Significant differences in terms of trueness were found comparing the 100 μm printing layer thickness to other groups. Therefore, the first null hypothesis was rejected. The best margin quality was found in milled crowns, followed by the 50 μm layer thickness group. Accordingly, the second null hypothesis was rejected.

In terms of trueness, the present study showed that 3D-printed interim crowns, printed with a layer thickness of 20 or 50 μm, are similar to the milled interim crowns, which are currently used routinely. Similar results have been reported also for 3D-printed ceramic crowns [15,35]. The effect of the layer thickness on the trueness of 3D printed casts and complete dentures has been demonstrated in previous studies [30,36]. Those studies demonstrated the highest trueness when a layer thickness of 100 μm was used, whereas the 100 μm layer thickness resulted in the lowest trueness in the present study. The main difference between those and the present study may be due to the nature of the objects printed. Neither casts nor dentures have as thin and tapered margins as crowns have, instead, they have large plain and round surfaces [36]. When the layer thickness is too small, discrepancies can occur, especially with such thin margins [30]. The combination of thin layer thickness and thin margins could also be an explanation for the fact that the trueness seems to be slightly higher in the 50 μm group compared to the 20 μm group, although this difference was not statistically significant. It should be noted that the aforementioned scoping review on complete denture fabrication included various studies [36], which applied varying settings for the 3D-printing, and therefore, the deviations in trueness may not be attributed to the layer thickness alone. A study, which showed that layer thickness did not affect the trueness of printed models when 100 μm was applied, still recommended the use of 100 μm layer thicknesses due to the economic advantages as the printing time is shortened [37]. However, the time factor may be less important when small restorations such as crowns are fabricated. Considering the effect of the layer thickness on trueness at thin surfaces such as crown margins [30], high layer thickness may be expected to result in low trueness, which was confirmed by lower trueness and marginal quality found with the 100 µm group in the present study. Although a previous study has shown that the marginal fit of 3D-printed crowns is within a clinically acceptable range, and that there is no difference between 3D-printed and milled crowns [38], significant differences in the margin quality were found in the present study. The marginal quality in the present study was evaluated by a 3-point scale instead of absolute values, indicating worse margin quality of the 3D-printed crowns irrespective of the layer thickness. Interestingly, the margin quality was not influenced by margin location in 20 µm and 50 µm groups, but in milled and 100 µm groups. The significantly worse margin quality at the buccal aspect of the milled group may be due to the slightly narrower preparation margin on the distobuccal side. During the milling process, defects may occur at thin crown margins [39]. Hypothetically, the preparation margin could also be the reason for the better marginal quality at the lingual crown margin in the 100 µm group. The lingual aspect of the margin preparation was the most uniform, which might have allowed the crown to be fabricated accurately even with the largest layer thickness of 100 µm. A large layer thickness might have a negative effect on the margin quality, especially with varying crown margin thicknesses. The fact that the margins of the prepared tooth were not uniform at all aspects is a limitation of the present study. Future studies are necessary to determine the effect of layer thickness on trueness and margin quality.

The reference data set can be recorded with a laboratory scanner, or more precisely with a high-precision optical or tactile industrial scanner [40]. However, because such scanners cannot be used intraorally, the reference data set was taken with an intraoral scanner. The intraoral scanner used has a software that enables immediate scanning of the fabricated restoration and the analysis of the trueness of the restoration comparing with the design STL. Adequate scan accuracy with the intraoral scanner used has been demonstrated in previous studies on single crowns [41]. Generally, intraoral scanners have demonstrated sufficient accuracy especially when scanning partial arches, as executed in the present study [41]. Since the reference data set was used to fabricate all crowns, potential errors during scanning would be expected to affect all groups similarly and therefore, can be considered negligible for its effect on the comparisons aimed. The trueness was analyzed by the calculation of RMS differences between the test and reference datasets. Calculating RMS differences is the most commonly applied trueness analysis in digital dentistry [42]. However, the effect of different software programs to calculate RMS values between corresponding datasets is not clear [43–45]. The influence of the build angle on the fabrication of 3D-printed crowns has been shown in various studies [14,18,25,26,29]. The build angle of 45° was used to print the crowns based on the recommendation by the manufacturer. A 45° build angle is similar to 135° build angle in terms of crown orientation during the fabrication, except that the 45° angle assumes a buccal crown orientation while 135° angle assumes a lingual crown orientation. The effect of build angle on crown accuracy when DLP technology is used was previously investigated and the highest accuracy was achieved when 135° angle was used [18].

Due to the pilot nature of the present study, no sample size calculation could be performed. The sample size was based on earlier studies, focusing on the 3D-printing accuracy [14,46] and enabled the detection of statistically significant differences in terms of trueness and marginal quality. One of the main limitations of the present study is that only one material was used for the fabrication of milled and 3D-printed crowns. Since previous studies have shown that the material has a significant influence on crown accuracy [47], the present study findings are not directly applicable to other materials. Nevertheless, the present study is the first of its kind indicating the influence of layer thickness on the accuracy of 3D printed resin crowns. The quantification of the marginal gap size was not performed in the present study. Since there was no difference between the milled and 3D-printed crowns when a layer thickness of 20 µm or 50 µm was used, a major difference in terms of marginal gap size would not be expected between these groups, however, marginal gap measurements can be performed in future studies to see how milling/printing trueness translates to marginal quality. The fact that the margin quality was only assessed by one observer is another weak point. Since the observer was blinded during the evaluation, it can at least be assumed that the risk of bias (e.g., by personal preferences) was minimized [48].

5. Conclusions

Considering limitations of the present study, it can be concluded that the trueness and marginal quality of 3D-printed interim crowns was influenced by the printing layer thickness. For improved trueness and margin quality for interim crowns using the applied materials and settings, a printing layer thickness of 20 or 50 µm may be preferable over 100 µm.

Author Contributions: Conceptualization, G.Ç., A.R.C. and B.Y.; methodology, G.Ç. and A.R.C.; software, G.Ç. and M.B.D.; validation, G.Ç., M.B.D. and B.Y.; formal analysis, G.Ç. and W.-E.L.; investigation, G.Ç.; resources, A.R.C.; data curation, W.-E.L., M.B.D. and S.A.-A.; writing—original draft preparation, M.B.D. and S.A.-A.; writing—review and editing, M.B.D., S.A.-A., M.S. and B.Y.; visualization, G.Ç.; supervision, M.S. and B.Y.; project administration, G.Ç. and B.Y., funding acquisition, none. All authors have read and agreed to the published version of the manuscript.

Funding: The authors would like to thank Laboratorio Innovando (Mexico City, Mexico) for their support in milling crowns and 3D Sequence Digital Laboratorio (Mexico City, Mexico) for their support in printing machine. The materials used in the present study were self-funded.

Data Availability Statement: Data available on request. The data presented in this study are available on request from the corresponding author. The data are not publicly available due to ongoing research using the data.

Acknowledgments: The authors would like to thank Laboratorio Innovando (Mexico City, Mexico) for their support in milling crowns and 3D Sequence Digital Laboratorio (Mexico City, Mexico) for their support in printing machine. The materials used in the present study were self-funded.

Conflicts of Interest: The authors declare no conflict of interest.

References

1. Liu, Y.; Ye, H.; Wang, Y.; Zhao, Y.; Sun, Y.; Zhou, Y. Three-dimensional analysis of internal adaptations of crowns cast from resin patterns fabricated using computer-aided design/computer-assisted manufacturing technologies. *Int. J. Prosthodont.* **2018**, *31*, 386–393. [CrossRef]
2. Kessler, A.; Hickel, R.; Reymus, M. 3D printing in dentistry-state of the art. *Oper. Dent.* **2020**, *45*, 30–40. [CrossRef]
3. Tahayeri, A.; Morgan, M.; Fugolin, A.P.; Bompolaki, D.; Athirasala, A.; Pfeifer, C.S.; Ferracane, J.L.; Bertassoni, L.E. 3D printed versus conventionally cured provisional crown and bridge dental materials. *Dent. Mater.* **2018**, *34*, 192–200. [CrossRef] [PubMed]
4. van Noort, R. The future of dental devices is digital. *Dent. Mater.* **2012**, *28*, 3–12. [CrossRef] [PubMed]
5. Dawood, A.; Marti Marti, B.; Sauret-Jackson, V.; Darwood, A. 3D printing in dentistry. *Br. Dent. J.* **2015**, *219*, 521–529. [CrossRef]
6. Muta, S.; Ikeda, M.; Nikaido, T.; Sayed, M.; Sadr, A.; Suzuki, T.; Tagami, J. Chairside fabrication of provisional crowns on FDM 3D-printed PVA model. *J. Prosthodont. Res.* **2020**, *64*, 401–407. [CrossRef] [PubMed]
7. Revilla-León, M.; Özcan, M. Additive manufacturing technologies used for processing polymers: Current status and potential application in prosthetic dentistry. *J. Prosthodont.* **2019**, *28*, 146–158. [CrossRef]
8. Salmi, M.; Paloheimo, K.S.; Tuomi, J.; Ingman, T.; Mäkitie, A. A digital process for additive manufacturing of occlusal splints: A clinical pilot study. *J. R. Soc. Interface.* **2013**, *10*, 20130203. [CrossRef]
9. Zeng, L.; Zhang, Y.; Liu, Z.; Wei, B. Effects of repeated firing on the marginal accuracy of Co-Cr copings fabricated by selective laser melting. *J. Prosthet. Dent.* **2015**, *113*, 135–139. [CrossRef]
10. Salmi, M.; Paloheimo, K.S.; Tuomi, J.; Wolff, J.; Mäkitie, A. Accuracy of medical models made by additive manufacturing (rapid manufacturing). *J. Craniomaxillofac. Surg.* **2013**, *41*, 603–609. [CrossRef]
11. Reyes, A.; Turkyilmaz, I.; Prihoda, T.J. Accuracy of surgical guides made from conventional and a combination of digital scanning and rapid prototyping techniques. *J. Prosthet. Dent.* **2015**, *113*, 295–303. [CrossRef] [PubMed]
12. Alharbi, N.; Wismeijer, D.; Osman, R.B. Additive manufacturing techniques in prosthodontics: Where do we currently stand? A critical review. *Int. J. Prosthodont.* **2017**, *30*, 474–484. [CrossRef] [PubMed]
13. Liu, Y.; Bai, W.; Cheng, X.; Tian, J.; Wei, D.; Sun, Y.; Di, P. Effects of printing layer thickness on mechanical properties of 3D-printed custom trays. *J. Prosthet. Dent.* **2020**. [CrossRef]
14. Shim, J.S.; Kim, J.E.; Jeong, S.H.; Choi, Y.J.; Ryu, J.J. Printing accuracy, mechanical properties, surface characteristics, and microbial adhesion of 3D-printed resins with various printing orientations. *J. Prosthet. Dent.* **2020**, *124*, 468–475. [CrossRef]
15. Lerner, H.; Nagy, K.; Pranno, N.; Zarone, F.; Admakin, O.; Mangano, F. Trueness and precision of 3D-printed versus milled monolithic zirconia crowns: An in vitro study. *J. Dent.* **2021**, 103792. [CrossRef]

16. Zhang, Z.C.; Li, P.L.; Chu, F.T.; Shen, G. Influence of the three-dimensional printing technique and printing layer thickness on model accuracy. *J. Orofac. Orthop.* **2019**, *80*, 194–204. [CrossRef]

17. Son, K.; Lee, J.H.; Lee, K.B. Comparison of intaglio surface trueness of interim dental crowns fabricated with SLA 3D printing, DLP 3D printing, and milling technologies. *Healthcare* **2021**, *9*, 983. [CrossRef] [PubMed]

18. Osman, R.B.; Alharbi, N.; Wismeijer, D. Build angle: Does it influence the accuracy of 3D-printed dental restorations using digital light-processing technology? *Int. J. Prosthodont.* **2017**, *30*, 182–188. [CrossRef]

19. Peng, C.C.; Chung, K.H.; Ramos, V., Jr. Assessment of the adaptation of interim crowns using different measurement techniques. *J. Prosthodont.* **2020**, *29*, 87–93. [CrossRef]

20. Peng, C.C.; Chung, K.H.; Yau, H.T.; Ramos, V., Jr. Assessment of the internal fit and marginal integrity of interim crowns made by different manufacturing methods. *J. Prosthet. Dent.* **2020**, *123*, 514–522. [CrossRef] [PubMed]

21. Simoneti, D.M.; Pereira-Cenci, T.; Dos Santos, M.B.F. Comparison of material properties and biofilm formation in interim single crowns obtained by 3D printing and conventional methods. *J. Prosthet. Dent.* **2020**. [CrossRef]

22. Mai, H.N.; Lee, K.B.; Lee, D.H. Fit of interim crowns fabricated using photopolymer-jetting 3D printing. *J. Prosthet. Dent.* **2017**, *118*, 208–215. [CrossRef] [PubMed]

23. Kim, Y.H.; Jung, B.Y.; Han, S.S.; Woo, C.W. Accuracy evaluation of 3D printed interim prosthesis fabrication using a CBCT scanning based digital model. *PLoS ONE* **2020**, *15*, e0240508. [CrossRef]

24. Davis, S.; O'Connell, B. The provisional crown. *J. Ir. Dent. Assoc.* **2004**, *50*, 167–172. [PubMed]

25. Alharbi, N.; Osman, R.; Wismeijer, D. Effects of build direction on the mechanical properties of 3D-printed complete coverage interim dental restorations. *J. Prosthet. Dent.* **2016**, *115*, 760–767. [CrossRef]

26. Alharbi, N.; Osman, R.B.; Wismeijer, D. Factors influencing the dimensional accuracy of 3d-printed full-coverage dental restorations using stereolithography technology. *Int. J. Prosthodont.* **2016**, *29*, 503–510. [CrossRef] [PubMed]

27. Yoo, S.Y.; Kim, S.K.; Heo, S.J.; Koak, J.Y.; Kim, J.G. Dimensional accuracy of dental models for three-unit prostheses fabricated by various 3D printing technologies. *Materials* **2021**, *14*, 1550. [CrossRef]

28. Çakmak, G.; Yilmaz, H.; Treviño, A.; Kökat, A.M.; Yilmaz, B. The effect of scanner type and scan body position on the accuracy of complete-arch digital implant scans. *Clin. Implant. Dent. Relat. Res.* **2020**, *22*, 533–541. [CrossRef] [PubMed]

29. Yu, B.Y.; Son, K.; Lee, K.B. Evaluation of intaglio surface trueness and margin quality of interim crowns in accordance with the build angle of stereolithography apparatus 3-dimensional printing. *J. Prosthet. Dent.* **2020**. [CrossRef]

30. You, S.M.; You, S.G.; Kang, S.Y.; Bae, S.Y.; Kim, J.H. Evaluation of the accuracy (trueness and precision) of a maxillary trial denture according to the layer thickness: An in vitro study. *J. Prosthet. Dent.* **2021**, *125*, 139–145. [CrossRef]

31. Park, G.S.; Kim, S.K.; Heo, S.J.; Koak, J.Y.; Seo, D.G. Effects of Printing Parameters on the fit of implant-supported 3D printing resin prosthetics. *Materials* **2019**, *12*, 2533. [CrossRef] [PubMed]

32. Schaefer, O.; Watts, D.C.; Sigusch, B.W.; Kuepper, H.; Guentsch, A. Marginal and internal fit of pressed lithium disilicate partial crowns in vitro: A three-dimensional analysis of accuracy and reproducibility. *Dent. Mater.* **2012**, *28*, 320–326. [CrossRef] [PubMed]

33. International Organization for Standardization. *ISO-5725-2. Accuracy (Trueness and Precision) of Measurement Methods and Results-Part 2: Basic Method for the Determination of Repeatability and Reproducibility of a Standard Measurement Method*; ISO: Geneva, Switzerland, 1994; Available online: http://www.iso.org/iso/store.htm (accessed on 22 December 1994).

34. Wang, W.; Yu, H.; Liu, Y.; Jiang, X.; Gao, B. Trueness analysis of zirconia crowns fabricated with 3-dimensional printing. *J. Prosthet. Dent.* **2019**, *121*, 285–291. [CrossRef]

35. Baumgartner, S.; Gmeiner, R.; Schönherr, J.A.; Stampfl, J. Stereolithography-based additive manufacturing of lithium disilicate glass ceramic for dental applications. *Mater. Sci. Eng. C. Mater. Biol. Appl.* **2020**, *116*, 111180. [CrossRef]

36. Vilela Teixeira, A.B.; Dos Reis, A.C. Influence of parameters and characteristics of complete denture bases fabricated by 3D printing on evaluated properties: A scoping review. *Int. J. Prosthodont.* **2021**. [CrossRef]

37. Dias Resende, C.C.; Quirino Barbosa, T.A.; Moura, G.F.; Piola Rizzante, F.A.; Mendonça, G.; Zancopé, K.; Domingues das Neves, F. Cost and effectiveness of 3-dimensionally printed model using three different printing layer parameters and two resins. *J. Prosthet. Dent.* **2021**. [CrossRef] [PubMed]

38. Haddadi, Y.; Ranjkesh, B.; Isidor, F.; Bahrami, G. Marginal and internal fit of crowns based on additive or subtractive manufacturing. *Biomater. Investig. Dent.* **2021**, *8*, 87–91. [CrossRef]

39. Li, R.; Chen, H.; Wang, Y.; Sun, Y. Performance of stereolithography and milling in fabricating monolithic zirconia crowns with different finish line designs. *J. Mech. Behav. Biomed. Mater.* **2021**, *115*, 104255. [CrossRef]

40. Pan, Y.; Tsoi, J.K.H.; Lam, W.Y.H.; Pow, E.H.N. Implant framework misfit: A systematic review on assessment methods and clinical complications. *Clin. Implant. Dent. Relat. Res.* **2021**, *23*, 244–258. [CrossRef]

41. Zimmermann, M.; Ender, A.; Mehl, A. Local accuracy of actual intraoral scanning systems for single-tooth preparations in vitro. *J. Am. Dent. Assoc.* **2020**, *151*, 127–135. [CrossRef]

42. O'Toole, S.; Osnes, C.; Bartlett, D.; Keeling, A. Investigation into the accuracy and measurement methods of sequential 3D dental scan alignment. *Dent. Mater.* **2019**, *35*, 495–500. [CrossRef]

43. Pellitteri, F.; Brucculeri, L.; Spedicato, G.A.; Siciliani, G.; Lombardo, L. Comparison of the accuracy of digital face scans obtained by two different scanners. *Angle Orthod.* **2021**, *91*, 641–649. [CrossRef]

44. Peroz, S.; Spies, B.C.; Adali, U.; Beuer, F.; Wesemann, C. Measured accuracy of intraoral scanners is highly dependent on methodical factors. *J. Prosthodont. Res.* **2021**. [CrossRef] [PubMed]
45. Son, K.; Lee, W.S.; Lee, K.B. Effect of different software programs on the accuracy of dental scanner using three-dimensional analysis. *Int. J. Environ. Res. Public Health* **2021**, *18*, 8449. [CrossRef]
46. Alharbi, N.; Alharbi, S.; Cuijpers, V.; Osman, R.B.; Wismeijer, D. Three-dimensional evaluation of marginal and internal fit of 3D-printed interim restorations fabricated on different finish line designs. *J. Prosthodont. Res.* **2018**, *62*, 218–226. [CrossRef] [PubMed]
47. Papadiochou, S.; Pissiotis, A.L. Marginal adaptation and CAD-CAM technology: A systematic review of restorative material and fabrication techniques. *J. Prosthet. Dent.* **2018**, *119*, 545–551. [CrossRef] [PubMed]
48. Day, S.J.; Altman, D.G. Statistics notes: Blinding in clinical trials and other studies. *BMJ* **2000**, *321*, 504. [CrossRef] [PubMed]

MDPI
St. Alban-Anlage 66
4052 Basel
Switzerland
Tel. +41 61 683 77 34
Fax +41 61 302 89 18
www.mdpi.com

Applied Sciences Editorial Office
E-mail: applsci@mdpi.com
www.mdpi.com/journal/applsci

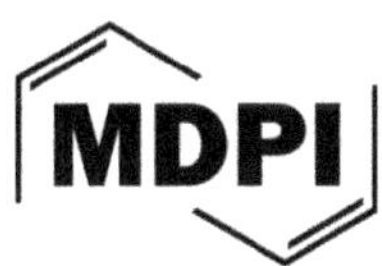